W74 ADV
(OWL)

Advances in
Health Economics

Advances in Health Economics

Edited by

Anthony Scott
Health Economics Research Unit, University of Aberdeen, UK

Alan Maynard
Department of Health Sciences, University of York, UK

Robert Elliott
Health Economics Research Unit, University of Aberdeen, UK

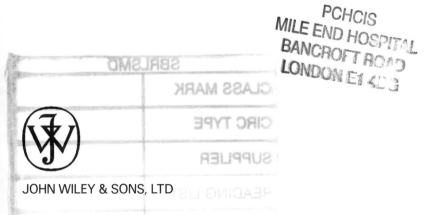

JOHN WILEY & SONS, LTD

This publication is designed to provide accurate and authoritative information in regard to
the subject matter covered. It is sold on the understanding that the Publisher is not engaged
in rendering professional services. If professional advice or other expert assistance is
required, the services of a competent professional should be sought.

Other Wiley Editorial Offices

John Wiley & Sons Inc., 111 River Street, Hoboken, NJ 07030, USA

Jossey-Bass, 989 Market Street, San Francisco, CA 94103-1741, USA

Wiley-VCH Verlag GmbH, Boschstr. 12, D-69469 Weinheim, Germany

John Wiley & Sons Australia Ltd, 33 Park Road, Milton, Queensland 4064, Australia

John Wiley & Sons (Asia) Pte Ltd, 2 Clementi Loop #02-01, Jin Xing Distripark, Singapore
129809

John Wiley & Sons Canada Ltd, 22 Worcester Road, Etobicoke, Ontario, Canada
M9W 1L1

Wiley also publishes its books in a variety of electronic formats. Some content that appears
in print may not be available in electronic books.

Library of Congress Cataloging-in-Publication Data

Advances in health economics / edited by Anthony Scott, Alan Maynard, Robert Elliott.
   p.cm.
   Includes bibliographical references and index.
   ISBN 0-470-84883-9 (alk. paper)
   1. Medical economics. I. Scott, Anthony, 1967- II. Maynard, Alan. III. Elliott, R. F.
   RA410.A48 2002
   338.4′33621–dc21

British Library Cataloguing in Publication Data

A catalogue record for this book is available from the British Library

ISBN 0 470 84883 9

Typeset by Dobbie Typesetting Ltd, Tavistock, Devon.
Printed and bound in Great Britain by Biddles Ltd, Guildford, Surrey.
This book is printed on acid-free paper responsibly manufactured from sustainable forestry
in which at least two trees are planted for each one used for paper production.

Dedication

This book is dedicated to Roy Weir, who together with Elizabeth Russell and Gavin Mooney founded HERU. It was, however, Roy's vision that was the true inspiration for the establishment of HERU.

Contents

List of Contributors

EMANUELA ANTONAZZO
Department of Economics, University of Bologna and Regional Health Agency of Emilia Romagna, Via A. Muro 21, Bologna, Italy
Email: eantonazzo@asr.regione.emilia.romagna.it

PROFFESOR JOHN CAIRNS
Health Economics Research Unit, University of Aberdeen, University Medical Buildings, Foresterhill, Aberdeen AB25 2ZD
Email: j.cairns@abdn.ac.uk

PROFESSOR DAVID COHEN
School of Care Sciences, University of Glamorgan, Pontypridd CF37 1DL
Email: dcohen@glam.ac.uk

PROFESSOR NANCY DEVLIN
Department of Economics, City University, Northampton Square, London EC1V 0HB
Email: n.j.devlin@city.ac.uk

PROFESSOR CAM DONALDSON
School of Population and Health Sciences and Business School, University of Newcaslte upon Tyne, Centre for Health Services Research, 21 Claremont Place, Newcastle upon Tyne NE2 4AA
Email: cam.donalson@ncl.ac.uk

PROFESSOR ROBERT ELLIOTT
Health Economics Research Unit, University of Aberdeen, University Medical Buildings, Foresterhill, Aberdeen AB25 2ZD
Email: belliott@heru.abdn.ac.uk

SHELLEY FARRAR
Health Economics Research Unit, University of Aberdeen, University Medical Buildings, Foresterhill, Aberdeen AB25 2ZD
Email: s.farrar@abdn.ac.uk

KAREN GERARD

Health Care Research Centre, Mail Point 805, Level B. South Academic Block, Southampton General Hospital, Tremona Road, Southampton SO16 6YD
Email: k.m.gerard@soton.ac.uk

PROFESSOR ALASTAIR GRAY

Health Economics Research Centre, Institute of Health Sciences, University of Oxford, Old Road, Headington, Oxford OX3 7LF
Email: alastair.gray@ihs.ox.ac.uk

DR DAVID HUGHES

Economics and Operational Research, Department of Health, Richmond House, Whitehall, London SW1A 2NS
Email: david.hughes@doh.gst.gov.uk

ANNE LUDBROOK

Health Economics Research Unit, University of Aberdeen, University Medical Buildings, Foresterhill, Aberdeen AB25 2ZD
Email: a.ludbrook@abdn.ac.uk

PROFESSOR ALAN MAYNARD

York Health Policy Group, Department of Health Sciences, University of York, Heslington, York YO10 5DD
Email: akm3@york.ac.uk

PROFESSOR ALASTAIR MCGUIRE

LSE Health and Social Care, London School of Economics, Houghton Street, London WC2A 2AE
Email: a.j.mcguire@lse.ac.uk

DR PAUL MCNAMEE

Health Economics Research Unit, University of Aberdeen, University Medical Buildings, Foresterhill, Aberdeen AB25 2ZD

PROFESSOR GAVIN MOONEY

Social and Public Health Economics Research Group, Curtin University of Technology, GPO Box U1987, Perth, Western Australia 6845, Australia
Email: g.mooney@curtin.edu.au

PROFESSOR DAVID PARKIN

Department of Economics, City University, Northampton Square, London EC1V 0HB
Email: d.parkin@city.ac.uk

PROFESSOR ELIZABETH RUSSELL

Department of Public Health, University of Aberdeen, University Medical Buildings,

Foresterhill, Aberdeen AB25 2ZD
Email: e.m.russel@abdn.ac.uk

PROFESSOR MANDY
RYAN
Health Economics Research Unit, University of
Aberdeen, University Medical Buildings,
Foresterhill, Aberdeen AB25 2ZD
Email: m.ryan@abdn.ac.uk

DR ANTHONY SCOTT
Health Economics Research Unit, University of
Aberdeen, University Medical Buildings,
Foresterhill, Aberdeen AB25 2ZD
Email: a.scott@abdn.ac.uk

PHIL SHACKLEY
School of Population and Health Sciences,
University of Newcastle upon Tyne, Centre for
Health Sciences Research, 21 Claremont Place,
Newcastle upon Tyne NE2 4AA
Email: p.shackley@ncl.ac.uk

DR DIANE SKÅTUN
Health Economics Research Unit, University of
Aberdeen, University Medical Buildings,
Foresterhill, Aberdeen AB25 2ZD
Email: d.skatun@abdn.ac.uk

DR SALLY STEARNS
Department of Health Policy and Administration,
University of North Carolina at Chapel Hill,
NC27599-7411, USA
Email: s.stearns@email.unc.edu

LUKE VALE
Health Economics Research Unit, University of
Aberdeen, University Medical Buildings,
Foresterhill, Aberdeen AB25 2ZD
Email: l.vale@abdn.ac.uk

DR MARJON
VAN DER POL
Department of Community Health Sciences,
University of Calgary, 3330 Hospital Drive NW,
Calgary, Alberta, Canada T2N 4N1
Email: mvdpol@ucalgary.ca

About the Authors

Emanuela Antonazzo is a Research Fellow in the Department of Economics at the University of Bologna and Regional Health Agency of Emilia Romagna, Italy. She worked in HERU as a Research Assistant between 1999 and 2001.

John Cairns is Professor of Health Economics in HERU, where he has worked since 1989. He is currently Programme Director of the Economic Evaluation research programme.

David Cohen is Professor of Health Economics in the School of Care Sciences at the University of Glamorgan. David was a Research Fellow in HERU between 1979 and 1985.

Nancy Devlin is a Professor in the Department of Economics, City University, London.

Cam Donaldson holds the PPP Foundation Chair in Health Economics at the University of Newcastle. From 1998–2002 he held the Svare Chair in Health Economics at the University of Calgary. He was Deputy Director of HERU between 1991 and 1998 and was Professor of Health Economics in the HERU from 1996 until 1998.

Robert Elliott is Professor of Economics and the Director of HERU. He has been Director since January 2002, and works half-time in the Department of Economics.

Shelley Farrar is a Research Fellow in HERU who joined the Unit in 1990.

Karen Gerard is Senior Lecturer in Health Economics in the Health Care Research Centre, University of Southampton, and Visiting Senior Fellow at the Health Economics Research Centre, University of Oxford. Karen worked in HERU as a Research Fellow during 1991 and 1992.

Alastair Gray is Professor of Health Economics and Director of the Health Economics Research Centre, Institute of Health Sciences, University of

Oxford. He worked in HERU as a Research Assistant and then Research Fellow between 1977 and 1982.

David Hughes is an Economic Advisor with the Department of Health in London. He worked in HERU as a Research Fellow between 1989 and 1992.

Anne Ludbrook is a Senior Research Fellow in HERU, where she has worked since 1983. She is currently Programme Director of the Evaluation of Health Improvement research programme.

Alan Maynard is Professor of Economics and Director of the York Health Policy Group at the University of York. He was an Honorary Professor and part-time Acting Director of HERU during 2000 and 2001.

Alastair McGuire is Professor of Health Economics at the London School of Economics (Health and Social Care), and in the Department of Economics, King's College, University of London. He worked in HERU between 1981 and 1989.

Paul McNamee is a Senior Research Fellow in HERU, and began working there in July 2002.

Gavin Mooney is Professor of Health Economics and Director of the Social and Public Health Economics Research Group (SPHERe) at Curtin University in Perth, Western Australia. He is the founding Director of HERU, and worked there between 1977 and 1986, and again from 1991 to 1992. He held a visiting appointment until 1997.

David Parkin is Professor of Health Economics in the Department of Economics at City University, London. He was a Research Fellow in HERU between 1982 and 1985.

Elizabeth Russell is Professor of Social Medicine in the Department of Public Health, University of Aberdeen (retired). She was involved in founding HERU, and has been closely associated with HERU until her retirement in 2002.

Mandy Ryan is a Professor of Health Economics in HERU. She is currently Programme Director of the Valuation and Implementation research programme. Mandy has been working in HERU since 1987.

Anthony Scott is a Reader in Health Economics in HERU, and is Programme Director of the Behaviour, Performance and Organisation of Care research programme. He joined the Unit in 1994.

Phil Shackley is Senior Lecturer in Health Economics at the University of Newcastle. He was a Research Fellow in HERU between 1991 and 1996.

Diane Skåtun is a Research Fellow in HERU, and has worked there since 1999.

Sally Stearns is Associate Professor in the Department of Health Policy and Administration, University of North Carolina at Chapel Hill, USA. Sally worked in HERU as a Senior Research Fellow from 2000 to 2002.

Luke Vale is a Senior Research Fellow in HERU, and has worked there since 1995.

Marjon van der Pol is Assistant Professor in the Department of Community Health Sciences at the University of Calgary, Canada. Marjon worked in HERU as a Research Fellow from 1995 to 2001.

Preface

In April 1977, the Health Economics Research Unit (HERU) was established in Aberdeen. It was the first research unit in the UK and Europe with a focus solely on health economics. The 'core' funding of HERU was from the Chief Scientist Office of the Scottish Home and Health Department (now the Scottish Executive Department of Health), and this remains the main source of funding for HERU more than 25 years after its inception.

In the early 1970s, health economists at the University of York had begun to establish a critical mass for the emerging sub-discipline of health economics through the establishment of the Health Economists' Study Group. Another key development in health economics occurred in 1974, when Gavin Mooney moved from the Department of Health and Social Security to the Department of Community Medicine at the University of Aberdeen for Scotland's first formal health economics project. The collaboration between Gavin Mooney, Roy Weir and Elizabeth Russell led to the establishment of HERU in 1977.

To mark the 25th anniversary of HERU, three events were held in May 2002. The first was a major policy conference held in Aberdeen, *'What can health economics do for the NHS in Scotland?'* The Chief Scientist Office and the Scottish Economic Policy Network ('Scotecon') sponsored this conference, which celebrated the contribution of HERU to policy and decision-making in the NHS. Presentations by HERU staff on the contribution of health economics research in the areas of benefit assessment, labour markets and health technology assessment formed the main part of the day, which concluded with a panel discussion on future priorities for health economics research in Scotland. The second event was a dinner, hosted by HERU's new Director Bob Elliott, where all current and ex-HERU staff (plus a few close associates) reflected on HERU's achievements and toasted the future. The third event had an academic focus and was a workshop to discuss the first drafts of chapters for this book. This was 'HESG' style and so involved a number of discussants selected from ex-HERU staff. The workshop was a successful conclusion to the 25th anniversary celebrations.

The purpose of this book is to reflect the unique and distinct contribution of HERU to the practice of health economics. Chapters have been selected to reflect a range of topics and methodologies in which HERU has played, and continues to play, a leading role. Each chapter focuses on the current issues and debates, and is forward-looking in terms of the research agenda and policy issues that are discussed.

The chapters are organized into four themes: methodologies (Chapters 1–4); performance and behaviour (Chapters 5–7); specific populations (Chapters 8–10); and equity in health care (Chapters 11 and 12). These themes trace HERU's contribution from a number of perspectives.

Methodologies. The development of methodologies is an important part of the development of any academic discipline and research in this area has underpinned much of HERU's work in applied health economics. HERU's contribution to methodology has been primarily in the area of valuation of the benefits of health care, arising from the need to be able to determine patients' and the community's preferences for health care. These issues are also relevant when considering equity in health care, a continuing interest of Gavin Mooney that is reflected in the penultimate chapter of this book.

Obtaining information on the value that consumers place on health care services is a key aspect of the demand for health care. It is necessary because of the severe market failures in health care which mean that prices for health care services and inputs, if they exist at all, are unlikely to reflect the value placed on these services by consumers. The development of non-market methods of valuation, as a mechanism for eliciting the preferences of consumers of health care, is therefore essential if the theoretical notion of 'consumer sovereignty' is ever to be realized.

A focus of HERU's research has been on methods of non-market valuation, which recognize that 'health' is not the only outcome from health care services that is valued by consumers. The development of the method of 'willingness to pay' (WTP) and 'discrete choice experiments' (DCEs) in health care, including their key methodological issues, forms the content of the first two chapters by Donaldson and Shackley, and Ryan and Gerard respectively. The key messages for both of these techniques are that considerable progress has been made with the development of these methods, and that further methodological work is required before these techniques can be used in the policy arena. The next decade will see both techniques more firmly established amongst health economists and policy-makers.

The valuation of future health events has also been a key methodological area in HERU's research. Such research aids understanding of individuals' health-affecting behaviour, as well as providing guidance on the use of appropriate methods of discounting in economic evaluation. In Chapter 3, van der Pol and Cairns compare a number of methods used to elicit preferences over future health events. They highlight issues with the validity of the stated preference methods being used, and conclude that comparisons with revealed preference data should be the focus of future research.

The valuation of benefits from health care needs to be incorporated into the framework of economic evaluation if they are to aid decision-making in health care. Getting the results of economic evaluations used by decision-makers is the topic of Chapter 4, by Gray and Vale. They report on the methodological issues involved to make the results of economic evaluations more useful and accessible to decision-makers. This is an important area if the research health economists undertake is to bear any fruit. The relationship between academic research, policy and decision-making is something that HERU continues to address, and much of its funding over the last 25 years has come from these same policy and decision-makers.

Performance and behaviour. Establishing what people want from health care given the resources available is a pre-condition for policies designed to change the behaviour of health care providers. Market failure in health care means that providers are not sensitive to the preferences of consumers. Research into the performance and behaviour of doctors, nurses and health care organizations therefore provides evidence about those regulations, contracts, payment systems and other factors that can be used to align providers' behaviour with consumers' welfare.

HERU's research in this area over the years has covered a number of areas, including agency in health care, supplier-induced demand, incentives for GPs, hospital objectives, nursing labour markets and the performance of health care systems. Three chapters in this book reflect this theme of work. Chapter 5 (Scott and Farrar) examines recent developments in the economics of incentives and agency, and how they can be applied in the UK NHS. It documents the reasons why explicit incentive schemes may not work in the complex reality of the NHS, and examines other ways in which behaviour can be changed, such as subjective performance evaluation, incentives in teams, bureaucratic rules, internal and external labour markets, and intrinsic motivation and social context. None of these have yet been examined in the context of the UK NHS.

As well as incentives to enhance performance and change behaviour of existing staff and health care providers, a necessary pre-condition is that there exist 'adequate' numbers of health care professionals. Elliott, Skåtun and Antonazzo in Chapter 6 examine behaviour in the labour market for nurses. Issues with respect to the supply and demand for nurses, including a review of empirical work, are presented and discussed. There are only a handful of studies in the UK examining these issues, even though this is a crucial area of health policy.

A focus on the performance of NHS organizations, in addition to the performance of individuals within them, has been the objective of ongoing reform of the NHS. The economics of hospital reimbursement is reviewed in Chapter 7, by McGuire and Hughes. The pursuit of efficiency in hospital production is considered, through the use of pricing rules, the consideration of the hospital as a firm, the determinants of hospital costs and scale, and incentives in reimbursement. The effects of reimbursement and regulation on quality are the main issues for future research.

Specific populations. HERU continues to conduct research into a wide variety of applied topic areas in health care that utilize a number of different methodological approaches. These topics may be defined in terms of a specific sector of the NHS, type of provider, type of clinical problem, or a specific population of patients. The three chapters here reflect some of the past, ongoing and proposed future applied areas of work in HERU.

Dental care is an area where there has been little work by health economists. Parkin and Devlin in Chapter 8 address the measurement of efficiency in dental care. This draws on a strong tradition of research in this area at HERU. Parkin and Devlin examine the nature of the commodity dental care, current issues in the economic evaluation of dental services, and the measurement of the performance of dental health care systems at a more aggregate level. The authors highlight the role of production function approaches to examine the determinants of oral health, and also note the scope for further research on the development of preference-based outcome measures.

The role of ageing and its effect on health expenditures has been a more recent focus of interest in HERU. McNamee and Stearns note the concerns raised by an ageing population on health care expenditures in Chapter 9. Their review of work in this area includes an examination of the relationship between age and disability, and age and expenditures. The jury is still out on whether greater numbers of older people in the future will be healthier than current cohorts. The relationship between ageing and health expenditures is complex and needs to account for the effect on social care expenditures. Further evidence, particularly from longitudinal panel surveys, is required given continuing policy changes in the area of long-term care.

A more longstanding area of work in HERU has been on primary care. Chapter 10, by Maynard and Scott, examines some of the key economic issues in UK primary care and general practice. Much of the recent reform of the NHS has given GPs and primary care an enhanced role in the allocation of resources. The main developments in the workforce, issues around nurse–doctor substitution, contracts, access and demand, and user charges are reviewed. The lack of routine data and a consequent evidence base for primary care reform has been a major barrier to the conduct of research in this area, which should focus on research in labour markets, skill mix and the role of the primary care team.

Equity and health. The final two chapters of the book are devoted to issues that are usually ignored by neo-classical economists who focus on efficiency of health care systems. Distributional issues and the role of determinants of health other than health care have broadened the scope of health economics.

The continuing work on equity by Gavin Mooney has led to new conceptual ideas about equity in health care, which are breaking free of neo-classical welfarism and highlighting the importance of community values that may be different from, and valued independently of, the aggregation of individuals' values. Mooney and Russell in Chapter 11 argue that these issues may provide solutions to the problem of allocating health care resources equitably across different groups, particularly with the notion of a 'constitution' for health services.

A focus of health economics research on 'health' rather than 'health care' is the key message from the final chapter by Ludbrook and Cohen. This reflects continuing policy developments, as well as the recognition that investments in interventions that influence lifestyle and life circumstances may have a greater marginal impact on health than investments in health care. Developing theory and gathering evidence on the demand for health, and the impact of these non-health care determinants of health, is therefore an important avenue of future research.

An inevitable outcome of the research presented in this volume is the identification of a complex and demanding programme of future research. The need for further research is as strong as ever, as the demand for health economics skills has increased in line with their supply (the direction of causality is perhaps an interesting area of research). Major changes in the structure and organization of health services, and advances in technology, will continue to shape the research agenda of health economics. Nevertheless, many research questions remain as relevant today as they were 25 years ago. What has changed is the development of health economics methods to address such questions more effectively, and an increased demand from decision-makers for the results of health economic studies to be used to answer key policy questions.

Anthony Scott
Alan Maynard
Robert Elliott

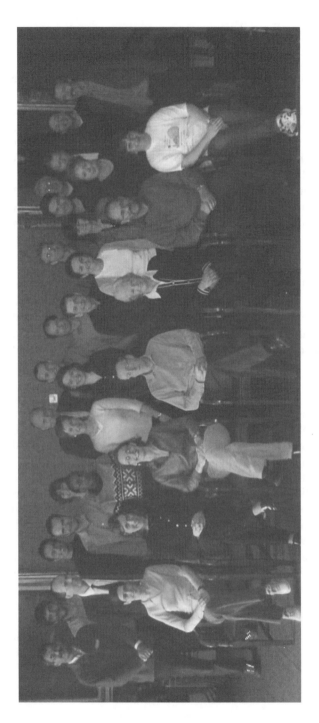

Workshop Participants

Front row from left: Patricia Fernandes, Emma McIntosh, Mandy Ryan, Bob Elliott, Elizabeth Russell, Gavin Mooney, Anne Ludbrook. Middle row from left: David Torgerson, Paul McNamee, Mary Kilonzo, Marjon van der Pol, Sarah Wordsworth, David Parkin, Janelle Seymour, Karen Gerard, Shona Christie. Back row from left: John Forbes, Kostas Mavromaras, Cam Donaldson, Julie Ratcliffe, Nick Bosanquet, Steven Simoens, David Cohen, Alastair Gray, Andy Lloyd, Alastair McGuire, John Hutton, Tony Scott, John Henderson. Participants not in photo: John Cairns, Nancy Devlin, Shelley Farrar, Divine Ikenwilo, David Newlands, Juan Perez, Ian Russell, Sally Stearns, Luke Vale.

Acknowledgements

The editors would like to thank those current and ex-members of HERU who participated in a workshop at the University of Aberdeen to discuss the first drafts of these book chapters. Thanks also to Laura Heatherwick for secretarial assistance. Thanks also go to the University of Aberdeen for hosting HERU for the past 25 years. The Health Economics Research Unit is funded by the Chief Scientist Office of the Scottish Executive Health Department. The views in this book are those of the authors.

1

Willingness to Pay for Health Care

CAM DONALDSON

School of Population and Health Sciences and Business School, University of Newcastle upon Tyne

PHIL SHACKLEY

School of Population and Health Sciences, University of Newcastle upon Tyne

INTRODUCTION

> 'Political economy has to take as the measure of utility of an object the maximum sacrifice which each consumer would be willing to make in order to acquire the object . . . the only real utility is that which people are willing to pay for.' (Dupuit 1844)

Although the concept of willingness to pay (WTP) has existed for a long time, it was not until the 1960s that the first empirical application was published in a journal (Davis 1963). This was in the area of environmental policy evaluation, and was specifically concerned with estimating the benefits of outdoor recreation in a backwoods area in the US state of Maine. During the 1970s, the method was further developed in studies of the valuation of human life, as applied to safety and transport policies (Jones-Lee 1974, 1976; Mooney 1977) and was first applied in the health area in the famous study of WTP to avoid heart attacks (Acton 1976). Subsequent to that, there were relatively few studies in the area of health (Diener *et al.* 1998), probably as a result of the quality adjusted life year (QALY) being perceived as a more acceptable measure of benefit than one which valued life in monetary terms. It was not until the publication of two empirical papers in the *Journal of Health Economics* in the early 1990s (Donaldson 1990; Johannesson *et al.* 1991a) and the conceptual paper by Gafni (1991) that the feasibility of using this method in health economics was once again recognized and more studies began to be undertaken (Diener *et al.* 1998; Klose 1999; Olsen & Smith 2001). In fact, Gafni was one of the few people to undertake empirical work in the health field

Advances in Health Economics. Edited by Anthony Scott, Alan Maynard and Robert Elliott.
© 2003 John Wiley & Sons, Ltd

during the 1980s, with his small study of the WTP of women on a kibbutz for contraception services (Gafni & Feder 1987).

There have been several advances in WTP methods during the 1990s. However, the contents of this chapter highlight the innovations with respect to designing WTP more in line with the welfare economic foundations of the technique and, consequently, making studies more relevant to decision-makers. Therefore, the chapter starts by focusing more closely on the arguments put forward in the early 1990s to justify the current resurgence of WTP in health economics. Three main sections will then follow. In the third section of the chapter, a perspective is offered on how WTP values should be used in decision-making. In this section, three substantive issues are addressed: how to design WTP studies to make them more relevant to decision-makers, given that values can be elicited from two groups (patients and the public) and for health care that is either publicly or privately financed; why WTP has not been adopted on a widespread basis in health policy environments; and how to account for the fact that WTP is associated with ability to pay. In the fourth section, the focus is on the progress in valuing benefits from the perspective of patients making choices between treatment alternatives (or close substitutes). This will be followed, in the fifth section, by a discussion of contributions in the area of using WTP methods at the level of eliciting values from members of the community at large with respect to priority setting amongst more disparate alternatives.

Before proceeding, it is worth noting that 'contingent valuation' is the more generic term for the kind of work discussed in this chapter, even though it is commonly referred to as 'willingness to pay'. The latter term is used here. While the focus of this chapter is WTP, it should also be noted that contingent valuation can also incorporate the estimation of willingness to accept (WTA) measures whereby respondents are asked what is the minimum amount of compensation that would be required for them to forgo a benefit or accept a loss. However, there are very few examples of WTA being used in health care evaluation. The most likely reason for this is that, contrary to theoretical expectations, empirical estimates of WTA tend to be considerably larger than WTP measures for the same 'good'. For a detailed discussion of the WTP–WTA disparity, see Duborg et al. (1994). Nevertheless, WTA should not be ruled out as a method of benefit assessment.

WHY WTP? WHAT IS IT AND WHY MEASURE IT?

WHAT IS WTP?

Put simply, WTP instruments measure 'strength of preference' for, or value of, a commodity. In areas of public sector activity, such as health care, in which conventional markets do not exist, decisions still have to be made about how best to use limited resources. This requires valuation of both resource costs of interventions and their benefits (i.e. health gain and other sources of well-being), the latter elicited in surveys by use of hypothetical WTP questions. In principle, with this type of information, the combination of interventions can be chosen which maximizes the value of benefits to the community.

It is important to distinguish WTP, as a measure of benefit, from the cost of a good. For any good, many people would be willing to pay more than its cost. Given that the good is provided at cost, and many would be willing to pay more, it is the maximum WTP for the good that represents its benefit to these individuals. For any individual, the difference between this benefit and the cost of the good represents a gain in well-being from having the good provided. This is why the concept of WTP is so important, and why the notion of *maximum* WTP was emphasized by Dupuit (1844).

WHY MEASURE WTP?

Shackley and Ryan (1995) outlined most of the reasons why WTP may have advantages over more general methods of eliciting community values, whilst Johannesson and Jonsson (1991) and Gafni (1997) have argued more specifically that WTP has advantages over other valuation methods, such as QALYs, commonly used in health economics. First, the questions used in many studies have been asked at too general a level, the paper by Bowling *et al.* (1993) providing a good example of this. Asking members of the public to rank alternatives as general as 'long-stay care' and 'preventive services' is unlikely to relate to any specific changes a decision-maker is thinking of making. Second, although the 'treatment of children with life-threatening illnesses' might come out top in such surveys, what is a decision-maker to do with such information? Services may already be in place to meet this priority. More likely, the priority will be partly met, the real question being whether more resources should be allocated to it at the margin *vis-à-vis* other potential service developments. Therefore, it is important to know how strongly other members of the community feel about proposed developments, not just about whom it would designate as more deserving groups. This is what WTP seeks to do.

Another advantage of WTP is that of 'getting beyond QALYs'. The QALY had been the dominant method of benefits valuation in health care through the 1980s, and remains so. In the following section, possible reasons for this are discussed. However, the potential of WTP was recognized as part of the debate about the limitations of QALYs which was also going on in the late 1980s (Loomes & McKenzie 1989; Mehrez & Gafni 1989). The 'getting-beyond-QALYs' part of the argument was that there are attributes of health care which may not be (adequately) captured by QALYs, such as non-health-enhancing aspects of the process of care and other consumption benefits like provision of information (Gerard & Mooney 1993; Mooney 1994; Ryan & Shackley 1995).

In principle, going beyond QALYs, by use of WTP, could aid in broader resource allocation decisions (e.g. between health and education). A final, more valid, reason for going beyond QALYs is avoidance of the separability assumption used in construction of QALY values; that is, the assumption that health-related quality of life can be separated off and valued independently of life years and other commodities is thought by many to be theoretically unsound relative to valuing goods more holistically (Bleichrodt 1995).

Despite these important favourable aspects, WTP has some outstanding (perceived) problems, these being the hypothetical nature of surveys in which values are elicited, how to use the numbers once values have been elicited, the fact that the method is rarely used in policy arenas and the fact that WTP is associated with ability to pay. It is research aimed at overcoming these problems which is reviewed below.

USING WTP IN HEALTH CARE DECISION-MAKING

DO HYPOTHETICAL QUESTIONS GIVE HYPOTHETICAL ANSWERS?

In studies of health care, of course, WTP studies are hypothetical with respondents being asked to imagine that they have to pay. This is inevitable, as not to do so would engender many 'protest' responses amongst respondents who would think that the exercise was about charging for health care rather than eliciting people's values. Furthermore, it might be argued that what is important in any decision-making context is the relative values derived for the options being compared.

Nevertheless, the extent to which values derived in such surveys reflect 'real-world' behaviour is an issue, influencing the perceived credibility of the method. In the early 1990s, the literature on this issue was split, with five studies showing WTP values elicited from surveys to be greater than those from real behaviour whilst five studies gave consistent results (Hanemann 1993). Since then, Carson et al. (1996) have shown in a systematic review of the literature that, compared with revealed preference methods, contingent valuation WTP estimates tend to be lower (on average 0.89 of revealed preference estimates), which is the opposite of what many people might expect. One study in the health economics literature has shown that a revealed preference and contingent valuation method arrive at similar valuations (Kennedy 2002), whilst others have shown the opposite to the Carson et al. review (Clarke 1997), with one also making the claim that it may still be possible to correct for any overestimation (Blumenschein et al. 2001).

Another major focus with respect to validity has been on scope effects: are split samples of respondents willing to pay more for greater amounts of the good being valued? Carson (1997) shows that most studies (31 of 35 reviewed) reveal sensitivity to scope. Despite such positive results, doubts still remain about WTP values elicited through hypothetical surveys. This has led to more qualitative methods being used to examine the thought processes underlying respondents' stated values (Schkade & Payne 1994; Chilton & Hutchison 1999), a trend which will likely (and justifiably) continue.

HOW SHOULD WE USE THE NUMBERS? THE PRINCIPLES

Despite the increasing number of WTP studies appearing in the literature, one important question appears to have been overlooked; that is how the results of WTP studies can be used by policy-makers. At first sight, the answer to this question may seem obvious since, conventionally, the decision as to whether to provide a service depends upon whether WTP values are greater or less than cost. However, the use of WTP values in such a way can be questioned, especially when, as is often the case in health care, values are derived from users of care (i.e. patients) and the budget for health care is frequently capped (Shackley & Donaldson 2000). In particular, the way WTP values are used will depend on from whom values are elicited (patients or the public), and whether the good concerned is privately financed or publicly financed through taxation (hereafter referred to as 'publicly financed'). This leads to four possible scenarios: (i) data are collected from patients for a privately-financed good; (ii) data are collected from the public about a privately-financed good; (iii) data are collected from patients for a publicly-financed good; and (iv) data are collected from the public about a publicly-financed good. Thus, it depends on the policy context. [There is, of course, a fifth possible scenario in health care, and that is where the intervention to be evaluated is a public good in the traditional economic sense. However, as is well known, public good characteristics of non-rivalry and non-excludability lead to problems in establishing 'true' strength of preference for such goods through the use of WTP. While there are examples of WTP being applied to public goods in health care, e.g. water fluoridation (Shackley & Dixon 2000), this fifth scenario is so rare in health care as to warrant no further discussion in this chapter.]

The conventional use of WTP values is encapsulated by Pauly (1995):

> 'The cost–benefit approach selects projects... by initiating all projects for which benefits are greater than cost, that is, all projects for which the ratio of benefits to costs is greater than unity.' (p. 109)

This criterion is acceptable provided that there is no fixed health care budget constraint. When health care is privately financed [scenarios (i) and (ii)], there is in effect no fixed constraint specifically for the good in question, since, if individuals are willing to pay for care (and if total WTP exceeds total cost), then premiums can be adjusted and the service will be provided.

Circumstances change once there is a fixed budget constraint for the good(s) under consideration, i.e. when there is a fixed budget to provide medical care services for a given population, even when total amounts allocated are increasing or decreasing incrementally. As Pauly (1995) notes, in this situation (which applies to publicly-financed goods as defined above):

> '...since costs are fixed by the budget, the general cost–benefit decision rule is to choose the set of actions with maximum monetary benefits.' (p. 106)

This is different from the conventional criterion of selecting all projects for which total benefit is greater than total cost. Thus, it is argued that the conventional approach is not appropriate when dealing with a publicly-financed good, i.e. scenarios (iii) and (iv).

With scenario (iii), the relevant constraint is the budget allocated to the treatment of specific conditions. In this context, it is the ex ante WTP values of patients which are relevant since it is patients who bear the opportunity costs of any decision and values collected in advance of care reflect preferences at the time a decision has to be made about treatment options. For example, suppose there are two alternative treatment programmes, A and B, which could be used to treat a particular condition. Suppose further that X patients have a preference for A and Y patients prefer B. The decision to implement programme A will mean that members of group X are 'gainers', while those in the other group (Y) will be 'losers' (the extent of the gains and losses being determined by the WTP values for each person's preferred over their less-preferred option). All else equal, the opportunity cost of implementing A is therefore the benefit that would have accrued had programme B been implemented instead. Clearly this opportunity cost is borne by patient group Y since they would have preferred programme B to have been chosen. Because it is patients who bear the opportunity cost of such treatment decisions, it is the values of patients which should be used to decide which treatment is implemented, all else equal. A method for doing this is described later in this chapter. If all else is not equal and the preferred treatment is also more costly, implying a potential expansion of the budget relative to other areas of care, this places the decision in more of a social context, as opportunity cost now impinges at another level whereby broader patient groups, each suffering from different conditions, would have to be compared.

This leads to scenario (iv), where the relevant constraint is the total health budget which is available to provide a whole spectrum of services. If WTP values are elicited in this context, it is the values of the public, rather than patients, which are more likely to be relevant since the public's values reflect the true opportunity cost context of decisions at this level.

Thus, at any one time, a public sector health care decision-maker will be faced with a number of proposals for expansion or introduction of services (say, A–D). Given limited funds, these proposed expansions would have to compete with some proposed reductions in care (say, E–H). What is important, then, is to obtain, through WTP values, an assessment from the community about their strength of preference for each of the options A–H. Although these options will inevitably be of different scales, and hence costs, the aim would be to choose that combination of projects which maximizes welfare (as represented by WTP) from the (marginal) funds at stake. Thus, it is not inevitable that A–D will replace E–H. Some of the latter may be retained. Empirical applications addressing this issue are described below.

USING THE NUMBERS: THE PRACTICE

There is a perception, which may be accurate, that WTP is not used much in policy-making. The simple response to this is that it is not problematic, because its validity is still being researched. Therefore, it is not ready to be used.

Another concern is that it is unethical to place a monetary value on the benefits of health care, and that this may be a view that is strongly held by decision-makers and others. Counter to this, however, the method has been used to help set priorities for provision of child health services in Grampian Health Board. The policy-maker, an employee of the Board, who was a co-author of the paper wrote the following passage:

> 'The view was taken that the WTP results were useful in summarising heterogeneous views, permitted opinions of the public to be investigated at a very detailed level and that examination of people's strength of preference added considerably to the understanding of their feelings about the health services concerned.' (Donaldson et al. 1997a, p. 22)

The method has also had a significant impact on raising the value of a statistical life used in cost–benefit analyses in UK transport policy and is used widely in evaluation of environmental policy and assessment of damage (Jones-Lee 1989; Carson et al. 2000).

There is little doubt that WTP suffers from a problem of perception relative to other valuation techniques. QALYs have received high-profile publicity in medical journals (Williams 1985). Furthermore, QALYs are perceived to be value free. Even some health economists themselves have stated their preference for an approach which 'considers outcomes equitably (as CEA using QALYs does), rather than to accept an approach in which choices are heavily influenced by ability to pay.' (Weinstein & Manning 1997, p. 127). For several years, the issue of distributional aspects of QALYs was largely ignored. However, it has recently been (theoretically) demonstrated that QALYs (and healthy year equivalents – HYEs) also suffer from the 'distributional problem' (Donaldson et al. 2002). Furthermore, it seems that the many criticisms of QALYs and how they are used in decision-making have been ignored by national-level bodies undertaking health technology assessments for approval of new therapies (Birch & Gafni 1992, 1994, 2002). Most of the people who write the guidelines to be used by such bodies are advocates of the QALY method. Guideline bodies composed of a broader range of economists have been more eclectic in the approaches recommended (Drummond & Jefferson *et al.* 1997).

Also, it should not be forgotten that, for decision-making within UK districts/boards (i.e. not at the level of national bodies, such as the UK's National Institute for Clinical Excellence), the impacts of QALYs and WTP have been equally minimal. However, this does not mean that potential does not exist. As an example, there is a perception that even a relatively unsophisticated priority setting mechanism such as programme budgeting and marginal analysis has not been used much at the district/board level. However, this perception has been recently contradicted by the evidence (Mitton & Donaldson 2001). Also, there has been no shortage of takers of the WTP method in studies evaluating different treatment options for patients (Johannesson *et al.* 1991b; Johannesson 1992; Johannesson & Fagerberg 1992; Donaldson *et al.* 1995, 1998a; Donaldson & Shackley 1997). These are mostly multidisciplinary studies in which non-economists, many of whom are health care providers, have to be persuaded of the value of WTP, often with no difficulty. To achieve more widespread use, however, a different dissemination strategy to the one (deliberately) adopted up to now will be needed. This will require more direct persuasion of policy-makers at all levels as to the value of the method.

THE 'DISTRIBUTIONAL PROBLEM'

A fairly typical view, and one that probably influenced the concentration of the health economics subdiscipline on the QALY in the 1980s, is that WTP should not be used in health economic evaluation because of its association with ability to pay. The implication is that WTP cannot be used where resource allocation is meant to take place on the basis of 'need'. A challenge to this view was apparent in parts of papers published throughout the 1990s (Donaldson *et al.* 1997a, 1998a). However, they are best summed up by Donaldson (1999a), who began by demonstrating that WTP cannot be used to make interpersonal comparisons across different categories of ability to pay as values elicited would represent not only strengths of preference but also differing marginal utilities of income.

On reviewing the literature, it was shown that, other than acceptance or promotion of the position that distributional issues are important, little guidance existed on how to deal with it in economic evaluations. The criteria by which 'good' and 'bad' distributions are to be gauged are not agreed – and most frequently not even discussed by writers in the field. The different views of major economic thinkers are displayed in Box 1.1. Three general approaches have been suggested. The first is simply to leave WTP values unweighted on the basis that the current distribution of income in society is judged fair (see quote from Pauly in Box 1.1). However, other analysts (see Dreze and Stern) would disagree with this (see Box 1.1). Currie *et al.* (1971) took the decision-making view, whereby values would be provided to decision-makers for them to judge the overall desirability of change. This view is supported by both Little (1957) and Mishan (1988), each of whom argues against the use of distributional weights, the main problem with such weights being how to derive them. Boardman *et al.* (1996) propose a compromise through the use of sensitivity tests, and it is this 'solution' upon which Donaldson (1999a) based a three-stage process for addressing the distributional problem with WTP. This solution allows the analyst to demonstrate the implications of using different weights without having to choose between them.

Box 1.1   Views of 'heavy hitters' on distributional issues

The Pauly view
'... if a dollar's worth of benefits to poor people were worth more to society than a dollar's worth of benefits to rich people, it follows that society should be redistributing income from rich people to poor people. If we observe, however, that society, whichever decision it makes, does not seem disposed to make further transfers from rich to poor, then we are not justified in asserting that the same society would value health benefits of a given money value more if they go to poor people than to rich people.

   To be sure, the analyst's personal preferences might involve more redistribution to the poor. But it is not legitimate to doctor the books in cost–benefit analysis in order to bring about by subterfuge what would not be tolerated in the standard political process.' (Pauly 1995, p. 118)

The Dreze and Stern view
'... at a minimum, one would want to see governments accepting some obligation to the weak or disabled.' (Dreze & Stern 1987, p. 958)

The Currie et al. view
"Describing the effects of an economic change on the individual groups is logically distinct from evaluating the overall desirability of the change. If the concept of economic surplus can be used to

describe the effects of a change, it has made a major contribution. Presumably, it is the responsibility of the 'decision-maker' to decide whether, on balance, the change is 'desirable'." (Currie *et al.* 1971, p. 790)

The Little view
"The conflict, which one may go through, between thinking that utilitarianism is nonsensical and thinking that there must be something in it, results from the endeavour to make it too precise. So long as it remains vague and imprecise, and avoids the use of mathematical operations and concepts such as 'adding', and 'sums total', there is something in it; but it becomes nonsensical if pushed too hard in the attempt to make it an exact scientific sort of doctrine." (Little 1957, p. 53)

The Mishan view
The Kaldor–Hicks criterion 'shows that the total of gains exceeds the total of losses and no more'. (Mishan 1988, p. 169)

The Boardman view
'... it may often be possible to use an approach that highlights the importance of the distributional implications associated with any policy being analyzed without requiring that any particular set of distributional weights be selected as the "correct" set.' (Boardman *et al.* 1996, p. 419)

The Harberger view
'The lessons from these examples is clear: When distributional weights are used together with weighting functions of the type most commonly employed in writings on the subject, the result is to open the door to projects and programs whose degree of inefficiency by more traditional (unweighted) cost–benefit measures would (I feel confident) be unacceptable to the vast majority of economists and the informed public.' (Harberger 1978, p. S113)

The first stage is to establish directions of preferences of individuals, with differing abilities to pay, for different treatment options. If the rich tend to have different preferences than the poor, this would be problematic. The second stage is to analyse the distribution, over treatment options, of strengths of preferences (expressed through WTP) across categories of ability to pay. This

Table 1.1 Distribution of preferences (mean WTP) [and number contributing to calculation of mean WTP] for location of delivery by income group

(a) Unweighted data

	Income (£s per annum)				
Preference	< 6800	6800–11,100	11,101–17,100	17,101–25,700	> 25,700
Labour ward	1	2	0	1	5
	(£200) [1]	(£50) [1]		(£100) [1]	(£1130) [4]
Midwives'	4	5	9	13	19
unit	(£67) [3]	(£415) [4]	(£240) [7]	(£238) [9]	(£250) [13]
No preference	3	5	7	9	5

(b) $X_i = Y_i^{-1}$

	Income (£s per annum)				
Preference	< 6800	6800–11,100	11,101–17,100	17,101–25,700	> 25,700
Labour ward	1	2	0	1	5
	(£575) [1]	(£80) [1]		(£67) [1]	(£542) [4]
Midwives'	4	5	9	13	19
unit	(£193) [3]	(£667) [4]	(£245) [7]	(£160) [9]	(£120) [13]
No preference	3	5	7	9	5

(c) $X_i = Y_i^{-5}$

	Income (£s per annum)				
Preference	< 6800	6800–11,100	11,101–17,100	17,101–25,700	> 25,700
Labour ward	1	2	0	1	5
	(£2009) [1]	(£27) [1]		(£1) [1]	(£1) [4]
Midwives'	4	5	9	13	19
unit	(£670) [3]	(£223) [4]	(£14) [7]	(£2) [9]	(£0) [13]
No preference	3	5	7	9	5

Table 1.1 *(continued)*

(d) $X_i = Y_i^{-10}$

Preference	Income (£s per annum)				
	< 6800	6800–11,100	11,101–17,100	17,101–25,700	> 25,700
Labour ward	1	2	0	1	5
	(£2190) [1]	(£2) [1]		(£0) [1]	(£0) [4]
Midwives'	4	5	9	13	19
unit	(£730) [3]	(£13) [4]	(£0) [7]	(£0) [9]	(£0) [13]
No preference	3	5	7	9	5

(e) Total WTP of those with a preference for labour ward and midwife-managed unit from four distributional assumptions

Weighted aggregation	Total WTP (£)	
	Labour ward	Midwife-managed unit
Unweighted	6,070	10,030
$= X_i/\bar{X}_i,\ X_i = Y_i^{-1}$	2,891	7,954
$= X_i/\bar{X}_i,\ X_i = Y_i^{-5}$	2,042	3,030
$= X_i/\bar{X}_i,\ X_i = Y_i^{-10}$	2,191	2,245

allows for detection of whether one group (particularly a high-income group) has the ability to distort average WTP values one way or the other. If necessary, the final stage is to undertake a sensitivity analysis of the effects of different distributional weights on the results of compensation tests.

Donaldson (1999a) applied all three of these stages to data from a survey in which women had been asked about their preference for one of two birth locations followed by a question asking them about their WTP to have their preferred option rather than that which was less preferred. Unweighted data on preferences by income group and WTP for each option within income categories are displayed in Table 1.1(a). The pattern of preferences across income groups is quite uniform. It should also be remembered that, in all groups, the second most frequent response is 'no preference'. There were no statistically significant differences in income between the groups preferring the midwives' unit or the labour ward. Generally, preferences appear to follow a stable pattern across income groups, although larger samples may have revealed statistically significant differences.

When examining strength of preference within categories of ability to pay (stage 2), the numbers of observations in each cell are small. However, treating the data as *illustrative* rather than definitive, it can be seen that, for location of delivery, the poorest and the richest groups are similar, with those preferring labour ward having substantially greater strength of preference. The opposite to this occurs in the three income groups between the lowest and highest. The strength of preference of those in the highest income group is not enough to reverse a compensation test in favour of midwives' unit care, but, potentially, could distort any decision about whether to have a mix of care instead of all one or the other. When data on medians rather than means are used, the result is similar.

Again, using these data illustratively, the method of weighting used in stage 3 is similar to that of Philips *et al.* (1989), the weights being inversely related to income. If Y_i is the income (before tax) of the respondent, a variable X_i can then be defined whereby $X_i = Y_i^{-n}$ ($n > 0$). Distributional weights can then be defined as $X_i / \bar{X}_i$, where $\bar{X}_i$ is the sample mean of X_i. Three values of n are used; 1, 5 and 10. The first of these assumes that marginal utility of income declines at a proportional rate, i.e. a person with 10 times the income of another will have their *marginal* pound weighted at one-tenth of that of the other person. With values of n of 5 or 10, the marginal pound of the richer person is weighted less than is implied by inverse proportionality. In addition, it can be observed where the critical value of n lies. The critical value is that at which total WTP for each of the options evaluated is equal. *Ceteris paribus*, a judgement could then be made as to whether the weights implied by such a critical value are acceptable. Thus, judgement by a decision-maker is still required. The results of the experiment with distributional weights are displayed in the remainder of Table 1.1. Given the rather draconian assumption in Table 1.1(c) that anyone with an income above £11,100 per annum has a WTP of zero, and that the midwife-managed unit still has a higher total WTP when this assumption is used [see Table 1.1(d)], it is safe to assume that, other things being equal, a midwife-managed unit is unambiguously the preferred option. The results presented here highlight the problems with such weights which have been pointed out by Harberger (1978) – see Box 1.1 again. When differences in weights are small, their influence on any evaluation is negligible and, when such differences are large, their effects can 'swamp' any efficiency considerations altogether.

As an endnote to this section, it is important to reiterate that QALYs have also been shown to suffer from distributional problems. Since all valuation methods use proxies to measure utility, it seems there is no escape from the issue that the value that is attached to the numeraire may vary across different social groups. But, hopefully, it has been shown that this does not hamper the usefulness of economic evaluation.

USING WTP TO VALUE CLOSE SUBSTITUTES

Many economic evaluations address the question of which type of care to provide for a given group of patients. These are the types of question also addressed in randomized trials. In the early 1990s, demand from other researchers for a WTP measure to use in randomized trials was based precisely on the need for something which 'goes beyond health'. Despite the potential usefulness of a WTP measure in such situations, however, the first problem faced is that WTP questions can be asked in at least three ways. The various methods, and their associated flaws, are outlined in the following section.

The first method is to ask patients who have participated in a trial comparing two types of treatment for their maximum WTP for the treatment they have had. Those having treatment A would give a WTP value for A, $V(A)$. Those having treatment B would provide a value for it, $V(B)$. This 'WTP for own care' approach was applied in a randomized trial of different antenatal screening methods for the detection of cystic fibrosis (CF) (Donaldson et al. 1995). In the trial, pregnant women had a CF carrier test (a simple saliva test) by one of two methods (i.e. disclosure or non-disclosure). Both parents have to test positive for the CF gene for a baby to have a one-in-four chance of being born with the condition. Under the disclosure method, a woman is tested, and only if she tests positive is her partner tested. The woman gets to know her own risk status. Under non-disclosure, both parents provide a sample and they are informed of their risk status *as a couple*. Unless a couple tests positive, women can never be sure of their individual risk status. This method is designed to avoid anxiety in women who, having tested positive, have to wait for their partner's test results before knowing whether the baby is at high risk.

Before receiving their test result, 176 women in different arms of the trial were asked what was the maximum amount of money that they were prepared to pay for the test. 127 women (72%) responded. Some were asked simply to state their WTP in response to an open-ended question whilst others used a payment scale. [The results of this part of the experiment were uncertain and are not reported here. Later research did follow up on this issue (Donaldson et al. 1998b), contributing to wider investigations into the validity and reliability of WTP methods by Johannesson (1992), Johannesson et al. (1993) and Donaldson and Shackley (1997), including assessments of the feasibility of eliciting WTP through discrete choice methods (Ryan & Hughes 1997) and comparisons of different econometric estimation methods (Donaldson et al. 1998c). These contributions, however, are different to the distinctive nature of the contributions which are the focus of this chapter, i.e. those paying more attention to the welfare economic foundations of the technique in the design of studies and, thus, making these studies more relevant to decision-makers.]

WTP did not discriminate between the screening methods. If there was a difference in utility between the methods, WTP, as structured, could not detect it. This result may have arisen because there is indeed no difference between the screening methods. However, this result has also arisen in similar uses of WTP alongside randomized trials reported in the literature (Johannesson & Fagerberg 1992; Ryan *et al.* 1997). It was reasoned, therefore, that in using such a WTP approach, individuals are likely to compare the care they have had with the alternative of doing nothing. If the most important thing is to receive some kind of test rather than no test, then it is likely that the groups will give similar WTP responses. A WTP approach which focuses the respondent on differences between alternatives may be more discriminating, suggesting elicitation of either:

1. a value for each alternative from each respondent (**'WTP for each'**); or
2. a value for one's preferred over one's less-preferred option (the **'marginal'** approach).

The WTP for each approach involves each respondent estimating $V(A)$ *and* $V(B)$. Making respondents aware of the choice to be made between a good and a close substitute in a sense recognizes the importance of 'reference points' used in prospect theory (Kahneman & Tversky 1979; Schoemaker 1982). Furthermore, data on respondents' preferences can be collected. A person's WTP for his/her preferred option can then be compared with that for his/her less-preferred option. Obviously, it is to be expected that the latter WTP is less than the former.

The study contributing data to assessment of the 'WTP for each' approach is the CF follow-up study (Donaldson *et al.* 1997b). Prior to an antenatal clinic visit, 450 women (who had not received one or other type of CF screening method) were given a questionnaire in which each method was described. From Table 1.2, it can be seen that most people preferred the disclosure method. The crucial result, however, is that respondents' preferences did not match their WTP values for the screening alternatives. 23% of respondents indicated either a preference for the disclosure method or no preference but were prepared to pay more for the non-disclosure method (see emboldened numbers in Table 1.2). The reason for this is that respondents' values were influenced by the perceived cost of each test; from one question asking about reasons for valuations, it was revealed that many women thought non-disclosure would be more costly, because they anticipated (erroneously) that it would involve twice as many samples as the disclosure method. Furthermore, it seems that the cost of the test was used as a basis for WTP; many women (roughly) estimated the cost of the test and stated that as their WTP. Therefore, *maximum* WTP was not elicited, which would raise questions about the validity of the approach.

Moving to the marginal approach, a value, $V(A-B)$, can be elicited directly. Respondents are asked to choose between the status quo (current care) and an alternative (experimental care), and are then asked what is their maximum WTP to have their preferred option instead of that which is less preferred. The

Table 1.2 Matching of preferences and WTP: CF follow-up study

	Is WTP (disclosure) >, = or < WTP (non-disclosure)?			
Preference	>	Equal	<	Total
Disclosure	62 (17%)	99 (28%)	**61 (17%)**	222 (62%)
No preference	1	22 (6%)	**21 (6%)**	44 (12%)
Non-disclosure	–	16 (4%)	78 (22%)	94 (26%)

Note: 90 people did not respond to the WTP question.

Table 1.3 Results using the marginal approach

Area of care and options	Number	Total WTP (£)	Mean (£)	Median (£)
Tonsillectomy				
Overnight stay (current)	39	1,119	43.08	27.50
Day care (experimental)	40	1,570	56.09	45.00
Midwifery				
Labour ward (current)	11	6,070	261.25	150.00
Midwife-managed (experimental)	57	10,030	263.95	100.00
Termination				
Surgical (current)	14	681	48.00	50.00
Medical (experimental)	34	3,350	103.00	50.00

aim is to try to make it clearer to respondents that it is their additional valuation of their preferred option that is required, regardless of whether the preferred option is more or less costly than their less-preferred option. The method also fits more closely with Kaldor–Hicks theory (Hicks 1939; Kaldor 1939). The simple rule provided by this theory is that a change should be made if the utility gains of those benefiting are greater than the utility losses of those who lose out from the change. WTP, using the marginal approach, approximates this theory by allowing the intensity of preference of those who would lose out from a change in care (i.e. those who prefer current care) to be compared with that for the gainers from such a change (i.e. those who prefer experimental care), assuming that costs are not under consideration.

Three studies have been conducted using the marginal approach to evaluate close substitutes amongst user groups (Donaldson *et al.* 1997a, 1998a; Gibb *et al.* 1998). The results of these studies are summarized in Table 1.3. As well as the technique being more discriminating (almost by definition), these results show that net benefits would have been substantially overestimated if the respondents had been asked to value the experimental treatment only. Furthermore, in two of the three cases in Table 1.3, the (apparently) less costly alternative, day care surgery in the tonsillectomy example and medical management of termination, received a higher mean WTP than the alternative option. This would appear to indicate that respondents are not considering cost when giving these valuations, but rather, as intended, are considering the extent to which they value their preferred alternative over and above that which is less preferred. In none of the studies did respondents indicate cost as a reason underlying their stated WTP value. Thus, the indications are that the marginal approach is more promising than either of the other two.

USING WTP IN HEALTH CARE PRIORITY SETTING

As indicated earlier, there are limitations as to how values elicited from patients can be used in decision-making. If interested in priority setting at the broader level, it would be useful to know if members of the population at large can compare disparate alternatives and express their strength of preference for each in terms of WTP. As mentioned above, an important role of WTP in this regard is in activating attributes in respondents' utility functions beyond health (e.g. preferences for equity in access). An opportunity to test the feasibility of such notions arose in an evaluation of a new helicopter ambulance service in Northern Norway (Olsen & Donaldson 1998).

Initially, the idea was to obtain a monetary valuation from the population at large for the helicopter ambulance. However, it was realized that, if such a service were to use up resources from a fixed public sector pot, then there would be an opportunity cost in not having other services available, or able to be expanded. Therefore, each respondent was asked to rank the ambulance service against 80 more elective heart operations for the community and 250 more elective hip operations. Each option was described in terms of who would get treated (e.g. men aged 50–60 years) and what the outcomes would be in the presence and absence of the intervention. The respondents were told that these options were competing for the same pot of money. After the rankings, respondents were asked for their WTP in extra taxation per annum for each option. The basic results are shown in Table 1.4, where it appears that helicopter and hearts are preferred to hips.

The most obvious fault of this paper was that, if hips were always asked about last, then perhaps respondents reached some kind of budget constraint (despite being told the options were competing with one another) or a fatigue level which deflated their final WTP (i.e. for hips). Thus, it would be important to test for ordering effects in the future. Other problems were that rankings implied by WTP often did not match the initial simple rankings given by respondents (Olsen 1997). Also, respondents were asked to express their WTP through taxation payments. However, at around the same time, suggestions had been made for taking more of an 'insurance-based' approach to WTP

Table 1.4 Results from Northern Norway study: WTP per annum (in NOK; $n = 143$)

	Helicopter ambulance	80 More heart operations	250 More hip operations
Mean	316	306	232
Standard error	25	25	21
Median	200	200	150

questioning, whereby respondents would get information on their own (or their family's) probabilities of needing care (Gafni 1991; O'Brien & Gafni 1996). This contrasted with the 'community-based' approach in Northern Norway where enhancements in programmes were described as being for the community (rather than using individual probabilities explicitly) and payments were through taxation. When asked why they would pay, substantial numbers of people mentioned altruistic reasons. A study published earlier, but undertaken after that in Northern Norway, in the field of safety improvements has shown, surprisingly, that valuations for private safety improvement were higher than for public safety improvements (Johannesson *et al.* 1996).

These problems and issues led to a project which gathered together a wider network of researchers around Europe who were interested in improving the method of WTP in the context of eliciting community values for priority setting. 'EuroWill', a project funded by the European Commission, involved surveys in six European countries (Donaldson 1999b). As well as addressing the issues listed above, the project has addressed several other issues which had arisen in the WTP literature during the 1980s and 1990s. These are listed in Table 1.5, along with other details of the surveys in each country. It can be seen that scope effects were tested for (through giving respondents different sizes of effect, in Portugal, and different numbers of people benefiting from the programme, in Norway). Also the payment scale was tested against the closed-ended method for eliciting WTP, the latter having been recommended by the National Oceanic and Atmospheric Administration of the US (Arrow *et al.* 1993).

The published output of this study has shed light on a range of issues in WTP estimation, including showing: the importance the population puts on community *vis-à-vis* acute services (in Ireland); the existence of ordering effects, reasons for them and, thus, potential solutions; the potential for improving consistency between rank orderings and orderings derived from WTP values by using an incremental approach to valuation, whereby respondents are asked for their WTP for their least preferred programme and then how much more (rather than absolute values) for their more preferred programmes; and that improved econometric techniques for estimating factors associated with WTP are required for surveys in which multiple alternatives are valued by each

Table 1.5 Issues addressed and numbers of responses in each country

Country (dates of survey)	Areas of care	Issues addressed	Numbers receiving different versions of the questionnaire	Total in each country
Norway (Mar 1997)	More heart operations More cancer treatments Helicopter ambulance	Insurance vs. community-based questions Size of effects	Community-based = 80 Insurance-based = 83 Community-based (two cancer programmes) = 79 Community-based (all programmes for less people) = 81	323
Portugal (Oct–Nov 1997)	More heart operations More cancer treatments Improved car ambulance	Numbers treated	Cancer, hearts, ambulance = 104 Cancer, hearts, improved hearts = 103 Cancer, improved hearts, ambulance = 103	310
Denmark (Apr 1998)	More heart operations More hip operations More cataract operations	Insurance-based vs. community-based questions Test–retest	Insurance = 168 Community = 168 Test–retest = 50	386
UK (May–Jun 1998)	More heart operations More cancer treatments Helicopter ambulance	Payment scale vs. closed-ended	Payment scale = 236 Closed-ended = 342	578
France (Oct–Nov 1998)	More heart operations More cancer treatments Helicopter ambulance Reduction in pollution	Process utility Cognitive capacity Test–retest	No process = 100 Neutral process = 104 Positive process = 99 Pollution/no process = 154 Pollution/process = 149 Test–retest = 50	353
Ireland (Apr 1999)	More heart operations More cancer treatments More long-term care	Marginal approach Ordering effects	Basic approach = 113 Marginal approach = 121 Different ordering = 101	335
Total				**2285**

respondent, and are possible to achieve (Luchini *et al.* 2002; O'Shea *et al.* 2002; Shackley & Donaldson 2002; Stewart *et al.* 2002).

CONCLUSIONS

Research on WTP in health care has developed substantially in the past 10 years, both on general issues of validity and reliability and on the use of WTP in the field of health policy evaluation. The research has:

- Shown the potential for survey instruments to produce valid measures of WTP;
- Produced a framework to guide the design of WTP studies in ways which reflect underlying theory and are more relevant for decision-making;
- Shown that, although WTP is associated with ability to pay, neither is this an impediment to the use of WTP nor is it a problem avoided by other valuation methods;
- Produced a more theoretically valid way of eliciting patients' preferences, which, at least initially, may work better than previous methods;
- Involved the conduct of the first survey where WTP was used to elicit strength of preference amongst members of the community for disparate options within a sector of the economy; and
- Created a European network through which several further methodological issues can be investigated.

An important advance from health economics has been to address whether the WTP method needs to be adapted for use in priority setting as well as in standard evaluations of care.

Important issues remain to be addressed, however. These involve experimental work to test methods of improving the consistency of results obtained in surveys combined with qualitative follow-up of survey participants to explore reasons for apparent inconsistencies and resulting possibilities for improving the survey instruments.

Given the amounts of resources at stake in health care globally, it is important to question continually, and to seek to improve valuation methods. The earlier arguments put forward in the chapter were outlined to help show how WTP was brought back into the research agenda of health economics to help with this, rather than to demonstrate its superiority over any other valuation method. With the jury still (and perhaps permanently) out on the issue of superiority, the health economics research described in this chapter has helped to establish WTP as one more method which economists can bring to bear in analysing complex resource allocation and evaluation questions.

ACKNOWLEDGEMENTS

Cam Donaldson holds the PPP Foundation Chair in Health Economics at the University of Newcastle upon Tyne. He is also a Canadian Institutes of Health Research Senior Investigator and Alberta Heritage Senior Scholar in the Department of Community Health Sciences at the University of Calgary. Thanks go to Julie Ratcliffe for comments on an earlier draft. The views expressed in this paper are those of the authors, not the funders.

REFERENCES

Acton JP (1976) *Evaluating Public Programs to Save Lives: the Case of Heart Attacks.* RAND Corporation, Santa Monica, Report No. R950RC.

Arrow K, Solow R, Portney PR, Leamer EE, Radner R and Schuman H (1993) Report of the National Oceanic and Atmospheric Adminstration Panel of Contingent Valuation. *Federal Register*, **58**(10), 4601–4614.

Birch S and Gafni A (1992) Cost effectiveness/utility analyses: do current decision rules lead us to where we want to be? *Journal of Health Economics*, **11**, 279–296.

Birch S and Gafni A (1994) Cost effectiveness tables: in a league of their own. *Health Policy*, **28**, 133–141.

Birch S and Gafni A (2002) On being NICE in the UK: guidelines for technology appraisal for the NHS in England and Wales. *Health Economics*, **11**, 185–191.

Bleichrodt H (1995) QALYs and HYEs: under what conditions are they equivalent? *Journal of Health Economics*, **14**, 17–37.

Blumenschein K, Johannesson M, Yokoyama KK and Freeman PR (2001) Hypothetical versus real willingness to pay in the health sector: results from a field experiment. *Journal of Health Economics*, **20**, 441–457.

Boardman AE, Greenberg DH, Vinning AR and Weimer DL (1996) *Cost–benefit Analysis: Concepts and Practice.* Prentice-Hall, New Jersey.

Bowling A, Jacobson B and Southgate L (1993) Health service priorities: explorations in consultation of the public and health professionals in an Inner London health district. *Social Science and Medicine*, **37**, 851–857.

Carson RT (1997) Contingent valuation surveys and tests of insensitivity to scope. In RJ Kopp, W Pemmerhene and N Schwartz (Eds), *Determining the Value of Non-Marketed Goods: Economic, Psychological and Policy Relevant Aspects of Contingent Valuation Methods.* Kluwer, Boston.

Carson RT, Flores NE, Martin KM and Wright JL (1996) Contingent valuation and revealed preference methodologies: comparing the estimates for quasi-public goods. *Land Economics*, **72**, 80–99.

Carson RT, Flores NE and Meade NF (2000) Contingent valuation: controversies and evidence. *Environmental and Resource Economics*, **19**, 173–210.

Chilton SM and Hutchison WG (1999) Do focus groups contribute anything to the contingent valuation process? *Journal of Economic Psychology*, **20**, 465–483.

Clarke PM (1997) *Valuing the benefits of health care in monetary terms with particular reference to mammographic screening.* PhD Thesis, Australian National University, Canberra.

Currie JM, Murphy JA and Schmitz A (1971) The concept of economic surplus and its use in economic analysis. *Economic Journal*, **81**, 741–799.

Davis RK (1963) Recreation planning as an economic problem. *Natural Resources Journal*, **3**, 239–249.

Diener A, O'Brien B and Gafni A (1998) Health care contingent valuation studies: a review and classification of the literature. *Health Economics*, **7**, 313–326.

Donaldson C (1990) Willingness to pay for publicly-provided goods: a possible measure of benefit? *Journal of Health Economics*, **9**, 103–118.

Donaldson C (1999a) Valuing the benefits of publicly-provided health care: does 'ability to pay' preclude the use of 'willingness to pay'? *Social Science and Medicine*, **49**, 551–563.

Donaldson C (1999b) *Developing the method of 'willingness to pay' for assessment of community preferences for health care.* Final report to Biomed 2 Programme (PL950832) of the European Commission. Health Economics Research Unit, University of Aberdeen and Departments of Economics and Community Health Sciences, University of Calgary.

Donaldson C and Shackley P (1997) Does 'process utility' exist? A case study of willingness to pay for laparoscopic cholecystectomy. *Social Science and Medicine*, **44**, 699–707.

Donaldson C, Shackley P, Abdalla M and Miedzybrodzka Z (1995) Willingness to pay for antenatal carrier screening for cystic fibrosis. *Health Economics*, **4**, 439–452.

Donaldson C, Mapp T, Farrar S, Walker A and Macphee S (1997a) Assessing community values in health care: is the 'willingness to pay' method feasible? *Health Care Analysis*, **5**, 7–29.

Donaldson C, Shackley P and Abdalla M (1997b) Using willingness to pay to value close substitutes: carrier screening for cystic fibrosis revisited. *Health Economics*, **6**, 145–159.

Donaldson C, Hundley V and Mapp T (1998a) Willingness to pay: a method for measuring preferences for maternity care? *Birth*, **25**, 33–40.

Donaldson C, Thomas R and Torgerson DJ (1998b) Validity of open-ended and payment scale approaches to eliciting willingness to pay. *Applied Economics*, **29**, 79–84.

Donaldson C, Jones A, Mapp T and Olsen JA (1998c) Using limited dependent variables to analyze willingness to pay data. *Applied Economics*, **30**, 667–677.

Donaldson C, Birch S and Gafni A (2002) The pervasiveness of the 'distribution problem' in economic evaluation in health care. *Health Economics*, **11**, 55–70.

Dreze J and Stern N (1987) The theory of cost–benefit analysis. In AJ Auerback and M Feldstein (Eds), *Handbook of Public Economics, Volume II*. North-Holland, Amsterdam.

Drummond MF and Jefferson T on behalf of the BMJ Economic Evaluation Working Party (1997) Guidelines for authors and peer reviewers of economic submissions to the BMJ. *British Medical Journal*, **313**, 275–283.

Duborg WR, Jones-Lee MW and Loomes G (1994) Imprecise preferences and the WTP–WTA disparity. *Journal of Risk and Uncertainty*, **9**, 115–133.

Dupuit J (1844) On the measurement of utility of public works. In JJ Arrow and T Scitovsky (Eds), *Readings in Welfare Economics*. George Allen and Unwin, London, 1969.

Gafni A (1991) Willingness to pay as a measure of benefits: relevant questions in the context of public decision making about health care programmes. *Medical Care*, **29**, 1246–1252.

Gafni A (1997) Willingness to pay in the context of an economic evaluation of healthcare programs: theory and practice. *American Journal of Managed Care*, **3** (suppl.), S21–S32.

Gafni A and Feder A (1987) Willingness to pay in an equitable society: the case of the Kibbutz. *International Journal of Social Economics*, **14**, 16–21.

Gerard K and Mooney G (1993) QALY league tables: handle with care. *Health Economics*, **2**(1), 59–64.

Gibb S, Donaldson C and Henshaw R (1998) Assessing strength of preference for abortion method using willingness to pay. *Journal of Advanced Nursing*, **27**, 30–36.

Hanemann WM (1993) Valuing the environment through contingent valuation. *Journal of Economic Perspectives*, **8**, 19–43.

Harberger AC (1978) On the use of distributional weights in social cost–benefit analysis. *Journal of Political Economy*, **86**, S87–S120.

Hicks JR (1939) The foundations of welfare economics. *Economic Journal*, **49**, 696–710.

Johannesson M (1992) Economic evaluation of lipid lowering – a feasibility test of the contingent valuation approach. *Health Policy*, **20**, 309–320.

Johannesson M and Fagerberg B (1992) A health economic comparison of diet and drug treatment in obese men with mild hypertension. *Journal of Hypertension*, **10**, 1063–1070.

Johannesson M and Jonsson B (1991) Economic evaluation in health care: is there a role for cost–benefit analysis? *Health Policy*, **17**, 1–23.

Johannesson M, Jonsson B and Borgquist L (1991a) Willingness to pay for anti-hypertensive therapy – results of a Swedish pilot study. *Journal of Health Economics*, **10**, 461–474.

Johannesson M, Aberg H, Agreus L, Borgquist L and Jonsson B (1991b) Cost–benefit analysis of non-pharmacological treatment of hypertension. *Journal of Internal Medicine*, **230**, 307–312.

Johannesson M, Johansson P-O, Kristrom B, Borgquist L and Jonssson B (1993) Willingness to pay for lipid lowering – a health production function approach. *Applied Economics*, **25**, 1023–1031.

Johannesson M, Johansson P-O and O'Conner RM (1996) The value of private safety versus the value of public safety. *Journal of Risk and Uncertainty*, **13**, 263–275.

Jones-Lee MW (1974) The value of changes in the probability of death or injury. *Journal of Political Economy*, **82**, 835–849.

Jones-Lee MW (1976) *The Value of Life: an Economic Analysis*. Martin Robertson, London.

Jones-Lee MW (1989) *The Value of Safety and Physical Risk*. Blackwell, Oxford.

Kahneman D and Tversky A (1979) Prospect theory: an analysis of decision under risk. *Econometrica*, **47**, 263–291.

Kaldor N (1939) Welfare propositions and interpersonal comparisons of utility. *Economic Journal*, **49**, 542–549.

Kennedy C (2002) Revealed preference compared to contingent valuation: radon-induced lung cancer prevention. *Health Economics* (forthcoming).

Klose T (1999) The contingent valuation method in health care. *Health Policy*, **47**, 97–123.

Little IMD (1957) *A Critique of Welfare Economics*. Clarendon Press, London.

Loomes G and McKenzie L (1989) The use of QALYs in health care decision making. *Social Science and Medicine*, **28**(4), 299–308.

Luchini S, Protiere C and Moatti JP (2002) Evaluating several willingness to pay in a single contingent evaluation: application to health care. *Health Economics* (forthcoming).

Mehrez A and Gafni A (1989) Quality adjusted life years, utility theory, and healthy years equivalents. *Medical Decision Making*, **9**, 142–149.

Mishan EJ (1988) *Cost–benefit Analysis* (Fourth edition). Unwin Hyman, London.

Mitton C and Donaldson C (2001) Twenty-five years of programme budgeting and marginal analysis in the health sector, 1974–1999. *Journal of Health Services Research and Policy*, **6**(4), 239–248.

Mooney G (1977) *The Valuation of Human Life*. Macmillan, London.

Mooney G (1994) *Key Issues in Health Economics*. Harvester, Wheatsheaf, London.

O'Brien B and Gafni A (1996) When do the 'dollars' make sense? Toward a conceptual framework for contingent valuation studies in health care. *Medical Decision Making*, **16**, 288–299.

Olsen JA (1997) Aiding priority setting in health care: is there a role for the contingent valuation method? *Health Economics*, **6**, 603–612.

Olsen JA and Donaldson C (1998) Helicopters, hearts and hips: using willingness to pay to set priorities for public sector health care programmes. *Social Science and Medicine*, **46**, 1–12.

Olsen JA and Smith RD (2001) Theory versus practice: a review of 'willingness-to-pay' in health and health care. *Health Economics*, **10**, 39–52.

O'Shea E, Stewart J and Donaldson C (2002) Eliciting preferences for resource allocation for health care. *Economic and Social Review*, **32**, 217–238.

Pauly M (1995) Valuing health care benefits in money terms. In F Sloan (Ed.), *Valuing Health Care: Costs, Benefits and Effectiveness of Pharmaceuticals and Other Medical Technologies*. Cambridge University Press, Cambridge.

Philips PR, Russell IT and Jones-Lee MW (1989) The empirical estimation of individual valuation of safety: results of a national sample survey. In Jones-Lee MW (Ed.), *The Economics of Safety and Physical Risk*. Blackwell, Oxford.

Ryan M and Hughes J (1997) Using conjoint analysis to assess women's preferences for miscarriage management. *Health Economics*, **6**, 261–273.

Ryan M and Shackley P (1995) Assessing the benefits of health care: how far should we go? *Quality in Health Care*, **4**(3), 207–213.

Ryan M, Ratcliffe J and Tucker J (1997) Using willingness to pay to value alternative models of antenatal care. *Social Science and Medicine*, **44**, 371–380.

Schkade DA and Payne JW (1994) How people respond to contingent valuation questions: a verbal protocol of willingness to pay for environmental protection. *Journal of Environmental Economics and Management*, **26**, 88–109.

Schoemaker PJH (1982) The expected utility model: its variants, purposes, evidence and limitations. *Journal of Economic Literature*, **20**, 529–563.

Shackley P and Dixon S (2000) Using contingent valuation to elicit public preferences for water fluoridation. *Applied Economics*, **32**(6), 777–787.

Shackley P and Donaldson C (2000) Willingness to pay for publicly-financed health care: how should we use the numbers? *Applied Economics*, **32**(15), 2015–2021.

Shackley P and Donaldson C (2002) Should we use willingness to pay to elicit community preferences for health care? New evidence from using a 'marginal' approach. *Journal of Health Economics* (forthcoming).

Shackley P and Ryan M (1995) Involving consumers in health care decision-making. *Health Care Analysis*, **3**, 196–204.

Stewart J, O'Shea E, Donaldson C and Shackley P (2002) Do ordering effects matter in willingness to pay studies of health care? *Journal of Health Economics*, **21**, 585–599.

Weinstein M and Manning W (1997) Theoretical issues in cost-effectiveness analysis. *Journal of Health Economics*, **16**, 121–128.

Williams A (1985) Economics of coronary artery bypass grafting. *British Medical Journal*, **291**, 326–329.

2

Using Discrete Choice Experiments in Health Economics: Moving Forward

MANDY RYAN

Health Economics Research Unit, University of Aberdeen

KAREN GERARD

Health Care Research Unit, University of Southampton and Health Economics Research Centre, University of Oxford

INTRODUCTION

Discrete choice experiments (DCEs) are an attribute-based stated preference valuation technique. They draw upon Lancaster's economic theory of value (Lancaster 1966, 1971) and random utility theory (McFadden 1973; Hanemann 1984) to examine the value of different goods and services by their constituent parts (or part-worth utilities) and by asking subjects to make hypothetical choices. Attributes of the commodity being valued are first defined and levels assigned to them. Statistical design theory is then used to construct efficient choice sets and individuals are presented with these choices in a context that is familiar to them. Analysis of the choice data allows estimation of the relative importance of the separate attributes, the marginal rates of substitution (MRS) between attributes and, if a price proxy is included, willingness to pay (WTP) for both changes in individual attributes, as well as changes in any combination of attributes. DCEs potentially provide richer information than direct WTP estimates by taking account of how component attributes impact on utility and use a less restrictive utility framework than the quality adjusted life year (QALY) paradigm, thereby allowing for consideration of attributes beyond health.

Advances in Health Economics. Edited by Anthony Scott, Alan Maynard and Robert Elliott.
© 2003 John Wiley & Sons, Ltd

Discrete choice experiments are being increasingly used in health economics. In a recent review about half the DCEs had been applied within a health economic evaluation framework, many to value dimensions of health benefit beyond health outcomes (Ryan & Gerard 2001). Other areas of application included: health insurance planning and premium setting (Chakraborty et al. 1994; Strensund et al. 1997), understanding labour supply characteristics and agency relationships (Vick & Scott 1998; Godsen et al. 2000; Scott 2000), extracting time preference values (Cairns & van der Pol 2000), developing prioritization frameworks (Farrar et al. 2000) and valuation of generic health status domains within the QALY paradigm (Hakim & Pathak 1999; Netten et al. 2000).

In what follows we describe the various stages of conducting a DCE in health economics, consider some of the pragmatic and emerging methodological issues that may be faced at each stage and suggest some topics for future research. We also give specific consideration to the issues of validity and generalizability.

IDENTIFYING THE ATTRIBUTES

The first stage of a DCE is for the analyst to define the relevant decision-making situation and the likely factors affecting choice of relevance to the commodity being valued. In particular the attributes of the commodity need to be defined. Attributes may be determined in a number of ways. If a particular policy question is being addressed then the attributes will be pre-defined. For example, if a health care provider is concerned with the trade-offs that individuals are willing to make between the location of a clinic and the waiting time or interest lies in different components of two arms of a randomized controlled trial. Where the attributes are not pre-defined preliminary investigations using literature reviews, group discussions, individual interviews and/or direct questioning of individual subjects will be necessary.

A *cost* attribute is often included so that WTP can be indirectly estimated. The direct WTP approach is associated with a number of problems, including lack of scope sensitivity, part–whole biases, status quo bias, cost-based responses, strategic biases, 'yea-saying' and warm glow (Ryan et al. 2001a) which the indirect approach may mitigate or avoid. It has been argued that the DCE indirect WTP approach may ease the task of estimating the value of individual attributes, overcome the problem of 'yea-saying' and incorporate built-in tests of scope sensitivity (Hanley et al. 2001). This is ultimately an empirical question.

An important question when deciding attributes is the question of how many attributes can be reliably evaluated in a DCE and what effect the number of attributes has on a respondent's ability to complete the choice task. Louviere *et al.* (1997) argue that increasing the number of attributes will not significantly affect results, although there is a consensus of opinion that DCEs should not be too 'complex' (Hensher *et al.* 2001). More research is needed to clarify what a 'manageable' number of attributes is; particularly as applications in health economics to date have included anywhere between two and 24 attributes, with a mode of six.

ASSIGNING LEVELS TO THE ATTRIBUTES

Once attributes have been assigned, levels must be assigned to them. These levels may be numerical (*cardinal*). For instance, time, distance, number of visits, in which case they are relatively straightforward to convey. However, often attributes are naturally *ordered* in some way. For example, when an attribute such as pain is described, it is possible to say that 'severe pain' is worse than 'moderate pain' but not that it is twice as bad. When levels are described qualitatively it is important to give attention to the description of qualitative attributes to minimize the ambiguity with which the levels are perceived, e.g. severe pain has similar meaning for all respondents. Attribute levels may also be *categorical*. That is there is no *a priori* assumption about which level is preferred to another. For instance, it is not clear, *a priori*, whether users of a service would prefer to consult a specialist nurse, a general practitioner or consultant. Pragmatically, the levels must be plausible and actionable, enabling the respondents to give the survey questions due consideration and also to avoid the raising of unrealistic expectations. They must also be sufficiently variable to estimate the parameters efficiently, which can mean levels set beyond current policy or practice level.

An important question when including cost as an attribute (such that WTP can be indirectly estimated) is the appropriate payment vehicle to use in collectively funded health care systems. At present the empirical evidence is just too scant to make a call. Most studies in health economics have used payment at the point of consumption. One study used willingness to accept (WTA) compensation (van der Pol & Cairns 1998), another (McIntosh & Ryan 2002) used travel costs and Jan *et al.* (2000) used a Medicare Levy. We need further exploration of alternative payment vehicles for applications of DCEs to collectively funded health care interventions.

A number of studies in health care have included time as an attribute, defining times in terms of waiting time, travel time, time to return to normal activities, duration of illness and time preferences. Interestingly, whilst most studies use a price proxy as the numeraire when estimating welfare gains, Ryan *et al.* (2001b) and Lattimer *et al.* (2002) estimated value in terms of time. Given that time is a commodity that individuals are used to trading in a publicly provided health care system, and it is measured on an interval scale, its potential use within the framework of an economic evaluation should be explored further. In the former study, a monetary measure of the value of time was estimated using the value of waiting time for public transport (Department of the Environment, Transport and the Regions' Highways 1997). This method assumes that the value of time when waiting for public transport is the same as waiting time in a health care setting. Such an assumption should be tested empirically and consideration should also be given to the relative value of the different types of time included in DCEs.

Economists have long been concerned with the value of reductions in risk and a number of DCEs have included risk as an attribute (Ryan & Gerard 2001). There is an implicit assumption here that subjects understand the way the risk attribute is defined. However, findings from the psychological literature challenge this assumption, arguing that individuals: view events as more likely if they are familiar; view hazards as more risky for other people than themselves; respond to risk information differently if presented in terms of either gains or losses or as a relative risk compared to an absolute risk; and code risk data in a categorical manner, i.e. 'low' or 'high' (Lloyd 2001). Wider literature ought to be considered when incorporating and defining risk into DCEs.

An important question when defining attribute levels is the sensitivity of the parameter estimates to the number and range of levels. Ryan and Wordsworth (2000) conducted an experiment to look at the sensitivity of the coefficients to the level of attributes. They found that whilst estimated coefficients were not significantly different across five of the six attributes included in the experiment, mean WTP estimates were significantly different for four of the five welfare estimates (Ryan & Wordsworth 2000). Within the marketing literature Ohler *et al.* (2000) found that whilst attribute range influences main effects to a small degree, substantial effects were found on attribute interactions and model goodness of fit. Ratcliffe and Longworth (2002) varied the number of attribute levels within a choice experiment and found that the relative importance of the attributes whose levels were varied increased as the number of levels increased, whilst remaining stable for those attributes whose levels did not vary. Future work should investigate this issue in more detail.

ASKING THE QUESTION

Once the attributes and levels have been defined the respondent is presented with a number of alternative scenarios that describe the commodity being valued in terms of different combinations of attribute levels. A number of different preference elicitation formats may be used – rating, ranking and choice-based exercises – but not all are consistent with an economic frame-work. For this reason our interest in this chapter lies only with choice-based exercises (although ranking exercises can be analysed in a manner consistent with economic theory, they have not proved popular with health economists).

The choice-based approach requires respondents to choose their preferred scenarios from a series of choices and the question can be posed in a variety of ways. If the *single binary choice approach* is used, it involves presenting individuals with a number of scenarios described in terms of the alternative attribute levels and for each scenario asking them if they would take it up, with possible responses being 'yes' or 'no'. An extension to this format, *best attribute scaling*, involves asking respondents, in addition to making a choice, to indicate which attribute they most and least prefer (Luce 1959; Szeinbach *et al.* 1999). This additional information allows attributes to be anchored by the least and most preferred choices and circumvents the problem of interpreting marginal utilities for attribute levels measured on different scales. It also avoids dependency of overall effect on individual attribute level scale values. A third approach is to present individuals with *multiple choice options*. Once again there are a number of ways of asking the question. Individuals may be *forced* to choose between two or more options (would you choose A, B, . . . , N) or they may be given an *opt-out* (the opportunity to say they would choose none of the options on offer or defer their decision). Alternatively they may be given the option to state their *strength of preference* for the alternatives posed (on a scale ranging from strongly prefer B to strongly prefer A).

There has been very little research comparing these different approaches and more research in this area should be encouraged. A single best approach is not anticipated, rather, better understanding is needed of the conditions under which different types of questions perform better. For example, *best scale attribute* questions may be particularly germane for studies that do not incorporate a common valuation scale such as money, risk or time.

EXPERIMENTAL DESIGN

A central part of DCEs is deciding what scenarios to present to respondents. The number of possible scenarios multiplies factorially with the number of attributes and levels. Rarely can all the scenarios generated be included in the set of choices presented to respondents. Experimental designs are used to reduce the number of scenarios in the questionnaire to a manageable number. Catalogues, computer software or experts may be used to do this. These produce a purposeful sample of scenarios for which values must be elicited to estimate a utility model.

The application of experimental design will be a function of how the DCE poses the question. If the *single binary choice approach* is adopted then all the scenarios derived from the experimental design can be presented to individuals. In the case where there are *multiple scenarios* within a choice set the resulting scenarios obtained from the experimental design must be placed into choice sets. This step raises the important question of how these choice sets should be constructed. A number of methods have been adopted in health economics, including: randomly allocating scenarios to choice sets; using one scenario as the constant comparator (could be the status quo) and pairing all others to it; or constructing a choice set that is orthogonal in differences between attribute levels (Ryan & Gerard 2001). Huber and Zwerina (1996) identified four principles which should be considered at this point: orthogonality; balanced design; minimum overlap; and balanced utilities. It is not possible to create a DCE which satisfies all four design principles simultaneously. Nor can the principles be applied in an unambiguous manner since there is no consensus for how to do this. Rather, the researcher needs to generate a number of choice set designs, check their properties with respect to these principles and select one, preferably with the most favourable properties. It is important at this stage to take account of realism as well as statistical properties of the design, and the researcher may forgo some level of orthogonality to select choices that are realistic.

ANALYSIS OF DATA

Response data are analysed within a random utility framework, using discrete choice analysis. Random utility theory states that whilst the individual knows the nature of their utility function, this is not observable. Utilities are therefore 'latent', and can be decomposed into a *systematic* measurable component and a *random* component. The systematic component includes the attributes of the commodity being valued (as well as other socio-economic factors that may be argued to influence choice). This is shown by:

$$U_{iq}(A) = vi_q(A) + \varepsilon_{iq} \qquad (2.1)$$

where $U_{iq}(A)$ represents the latent utility of individual q for good i with attributes A, $vi_q(A)$ represents the measurable component of utility estimated empirically, with i, q and A as defined above, and ε reflects the unobservable factors. Given that the researcher cannot observe $U_{iq}(A)$, but only $vi_q(A)$, the researcher can only predict the probability that individual q will choose good i from the total choice set. Assuming a choice between i and j:

$$P(i_q|A,C) = P[(vi_q + \varepsilon_{iq}) > (vj_q + \varepsilon_{jq})] \qquad (2.2)$$

where P represents the probability, C the total choice set (i and j in this example), and all other terms are defined above. For purposes of empirical measurement, a probability distribution is assumed for ε_{jq} and ε_{iq}, the random component.

When analysing the data assumptions must be made about the functional form of the observable indirect utility function (vi_q). Most applications assume an additive linear relationship between choice and the attributes included in the study. The additive assumption implies that there are no significant interactions between attributes and that the effects of the attributes on choice do not change as the level of that attribute changes, i.e. each unit change in an attribute has a constant marginal effect on choice. Despite evidence from outside health economics that main effects explain over 80% of the preference structure (Pearmain *et al.* 1991), the problem with (health) economic theory is that very often there is little *a priori* guidance for researchers on what interactions or higher-order effects should be considered in a design. Selected two-way interactions, in particular, may be sufficiently important to be included if they are expected to be as, or more, significant than an individual main effect in explaining model variance. To ignore these effects or pay insufficient attention to them will undermine the model. Focus on main effects plans mirrors past practice in the environmental economics literature, but here the view is changing and it would be apposite for health economists to keep apace of these developments (Adamowicz 2001). Such modelling needs to be built into the experimental design of the study, and requires data to be collected on a larger choice set.

Having decided the functional form of the utility function, the response data is analysed. The appropriate technique will depend on what method was used to collect the data. Given that multiple observations are obtained from respondents, random effects probit or logit models have been applied for binary choices. Where respondents are asked to evaluate more than two alternatives within a choice set, conditional logit or probit models should be used. Given that conditional logit is computationally easier, it is the most commonly used technique. It should be noted that such models are known to be subject to violations of the irrelevance of independent alternatives (IIA) assumption. This condition requires that the ratio of probabilities for any two alternatives be independent of the attribute levels in the third alternative. Violations of this assumption result in biased parameter estimates. Further, conditional logit models currently do not account for multiple observations from individuals. Nested logit models may be used to deal partially with the IIA assumption, though such models currently do not account for multiple observations from individuals. Random parameter logit may also be applied to discrete choice data sets (Revelt & Train 1998). This technique is not subject to the IIA assumption, takes account of multiple observations from individuals and allows for heterogeneity of tastes across individuals. Johnson *et al.* (2000) has used this method and more studies should consider it.

For ease of illustration in what follows we will assume a linear utility function (as is most commonly done). The researcher then estimates the following indirect utility function with the appropriate regression model (as defined above):

$$v = \chi_0 + \sum \chi_n X_n + \cdots + \delta P + \theta \tag{2.3}$$

where χ_0, χ_n and δ are the parameters of the model to be estimated, X_n represents the level of the n attributes of the commodity being valued ($n - 1, 2, \ldots, k$), $\sum \chi_n X_n$ represents the summation of all the model effect coefficients, P is the price level (or some proxy for price), and θ the unobservable error term for the model. χ_0 reflects the subject's preferences for one commodity over another when all attributes in the model are the same [referred to in the literature as the alternative specific constant (ASC), most likely to be important in 'labelled' DCEs]. The χ parameters are equal to the marginal utilities of the given attributes (i.e. $\partial v / \partial X_k = \chi_k$), and the ratio of any two parameters shows the marginal rates of substitution between attributes. Following on from this, the ratio of any given attribute to the absolute parameter on the price attribute shows how much money an individual is willing to pay for a unit change in that attribute (i.e. χ_n / δ). From this it is possible to estimate overall WTP for a change in the provision of a service by summing the product of attribute coefficients and their independent variables (i.e. $\sum \chi_n X_n$) and dividing by the absolute parameter on the price – the measure commonly used to estimate the welfare impact of a change in policy is given by:

$$\text{WTP} = \left\{ \left(\sum \chi_n X_n \right) / \delta \right\} \tag{2.4}$$

VALIDITY OF RESPONSES

It is important to include tests of validity, i.e. to test the extent to which individuals behave in real settings as they state they would. Given that many of the applications of DCEs have taken place in countries with a publicly provided health care system, and there is therefore a lack of secondary data sets to compare real and stated behaviour, a number of alternative validity tests have been applied. Current practice indicates that the most commonly considered notion is theoretical (internal) validity. This involves checking that model coefficients have the signs expected given theory or previous evidence. The evidence generally on the theoretical validity of DCEs is encouraging (Ryan & Gerard 2001). More recently, assessment of validity has given consideration to testing the underlying axioms of DCEs. In what follows we consider this growing literature. Finally we comment on the importance of conducting tests of external validity, the issue of strategic behaviour and the role of face validity.

COMPLETENESS OF PREFERENCES

Experiments concerned with modelling individual preferences are based on the assumption of completeness, i.e. it is assumed that individuals have well-defined preferences for any choice they are presented with. However, this may not be the case for goods such as health care, where individuals are not used to making choices. If this assumption is violated, the large body of experimental economic literature eliciting patient preferences in health care may be challenged. Research is at an early stage. Ryan and San Miguel (2002) report the results of the first DCE to examine the assumption of complete preferences within health care. The tests carried out were based on the comparison of preferences for three different goods for which different levels of formed preferences are expected: a supermarket, dentist consultation (chosen as a likely familiar health service) and bowel cancer screening (chosen as a likely unfamiliar health service). Evidence of completeness of preferences for all three goods was provided. Further evidence showed limited evidence of incomplete preferences when applied in a study of emergency health services (Gerard 2002).

RATIONALITY OF RESPONSES

For responses to be considered rational the individual should prefer more of a good thing rather than less of it. Dominance or non-satiation tests (i.e. choice sets where one alternative is clearly superior) are the most commonly applied rationality tests. It may be argued that dominance tests both challenge the credibility of DCEs (since some of the choices presented are so obviously 'superior' that subjects may think they are being tricked) and that they are 'easy' to pass. It has been recommended that alternative definitions of rationality be explored. More stringent tests have been applied to a few studies (McIntosh & Ryan 2002; San Miguel 2002) but this needs to be taken a step further and researched in conjunction with reasons for 'irrational responses'. Despite a growing literature from both psychology and economics indicating that apparently 'irrational' responses can be rationally explained (Loomes & Sugden 1992; Fischer & Hawkins 1993), there has been little cross-fertilization so far with DCEs in health economics. In future work 'irrational' responses should be explored with the help of qualitative research techniques (Schkade & Payne 1994).

CONTINUITY OF PREFERENCES

Estimation of a latent utility function implies that individuals have continuous preferences. It is from this assumption that marginal rates of substitution can be estimated. A number of issues are raised here. The first concerns current methods of testing for continuous preferences. To date DCEs have attempted to do this by testing whether individuals always choose an option with the 'best' level of a given attribute, i.e. whether they have dominant preferences. For example, if respondents always choose the option with the best level for a particular attribute it is concluded that they are dominant with respect to this attribute. The implication here is that such a preference structure is inconsistent with a continuous utility function. However, this may not be the case as it is possible to find more complex preference structures which are consistent with a continuous utility function (Ryan & Gerard 2001).

This does not suggest that all preference structures are continuous, but rather that current continuity tests within DCEs are incapable of identifying violations of the continuity axiom. Given the possibility of identifying some continuous utility function for all possible responses, alternative continuity tests are required. Work in this area may also consider the use of qualitative research techniques to explore decision-making strategies employed when responding to DCEs. Ryan *et al.* (2002) found the 'think aloud' qualitative research technique to be very informative when investigating the economics axioms of both continuity and rationality.

If non-compensatory decision-making is identified, questions are raised concerning the analysis of the response data. Whilst it seems to be generally recognized that under certain circumstances individuals may adopt non-compensatory decision-making strategies, to date compensatory modelling dictates. This probably reflects the modelling difficulties that would result from relaxing the assumption. However, recently Swait (2001) has developed a formal model for analysing a wide range of decision strategies that relax the assumption of compensatory decision-making. One anticipates that in future work this advancement will become increasingly important for appropriate modelling of health care utility functions.

One general issue concerning testing validity via the theoretical axioms is the relationship between complexity of the choice task and satisfaction of the axioms. Rational choice theorists would argue that the description of the choice set would not influence responses. Respondents to DCEs are therefore assumed to be able to respond to choice tasks optimally, regardless of the number of attributes, levels and choices. Whilst a limited number of economists have questioned this issue (Heiner 1983; De Palma *et al.* 1994), psychology has been more challenging of this assumption that task complexity would not influence the ability to optimize (Payne *et al.* 1993). Simon (1955) argued that individuals might adopt 'satisficing' decision rules, considering only a limited amount of the information available. As complexity increases, so would reliance on simple decision-making strategies. Heiner (1983) argues that as complexity increases, individuals will find the benefits of adopting simple decision-making heuristics outweigh the costs. However, such behaviour is not utility-maximizing. The psychology literature also indicates that respondents often employ simplifying heuristics in decision-making, employing 'fast and frugal heuristics' (Gigerenzer & Todd 1999). Such decision-making heuristics may also explain apparent irrationalities (Kahneman *et al.* 1982). It is necessary to explore how satisfaction of the economic axioms is related to complexity of the choice task. Findings here will also have implications for the experimental design of the DCE.

EXTERNAL VALIDITY

The preferred test of validity is whether individuals behave in the real world as they state in the DCE. No studies so far have tested this in health economics. The environmental economics literature has also focused on internal validity, with only one study carrying out a direct comparison of real and actual WTP (Carlsson & Martinnsson 2002). They found that DCE estimates of values for wildlife protection were insignificantly different from real payment obtained in an experimental setting. Health economists clearly need to attempt to apply tests of external validity [as they are attempting to do in the direct willingness to pay literature, see Blumenschein *et al.* (2001) and Clark (2002)]. Consideration should be given here to setting up an experiment to compare real and stated behaviour, or identifying secondary data sets where information on actual behaviour exists. Possibilities in predominantly publicly funded health services include those parts of the health care system that require co-payment, such as, in the UK, the demand for prescriptions, dental care or assisted reproductive techniques. An alternative would be to go back to respondents with the results from a DCE, and ask them if the results are consistent with their preferences. Future work should also explore the fusion of stated preference and revealed preference data.

STRATEGIC BEHAVIOUR

A closely related matter is the opportunity for respondents to act strategically. That is, to what extent can the respondent behave to influence the outcome of the experiment? Or has the DCE been designed in such a way to ameliorate this, encouraging the respondent to complete the DCE questionnaire honestly? These issues need to be given careful attention at the stages of survey design and data collection, and it would be extremely useful to report empirical findings from specifically designed tests in this area. Furthermore it will be important to comment on the incentive compatibility of studies (i.e. what mechanisms are in place to promote 'truthful' responses). To date these issues remain notable for their absence of empirics.

FACE VALIDITY

For DCEs to claim to be a validated technique evidence of face validity is also needed as this addresses the confidence placed in the DCE measuring what is intended by the researcher. Face validity is essentially a qualitative judgement and has not been highly visible in the current health economics DCE literature reported, although some studies have made endeavours towards it. To date there is no agreed-upon definition of face validity for DCEs but as the analyst is responsible for designing a DCE that closely models indirect utility and does so by exerting considerable control over many of the steps in the methods, it seems pertinent to draw out some of the finer detail in order to accumulate evidence of face validity. In particular, it is important that the researcher can justify: the most appropriate decision-making context has been selected for the study; key stakeholders have been involved in the process of defining and selecting attributes and levels; alternative ways to ask the choice question have been assessed; contextual information has been provided to respondents in a comprehensible form; and contextual variables and interaction terms identified *a priori*. Some of these criteria can be assessed by qualitative interviews, others are part of an analysis plan. Further evidence can be obtained by reporting whether (and how many) iterative processes were used to develop the final survey instrument; indicating an analyst mindful of minimizing random error and maximizing responses. We would recommend greater attention be paid to the issue of face validity in future studies.

GENERALIZABILITY

Health economics is concerned with the efficient allocation of scarce health care resources. Preference elicitation techniques, such as DCEs, are developed to help inform this debate. Preference elicitation experiments, whether they be standard gamble, time trade-off, willingness to pay or DCEs are often time-consuming and expensive to carry out. Given this, there has been an increasing interest in health economics in developing generalizable benefit measures which can be applied in a number of different contexts and settings, e.g. EQ-5D to measure the value of alternative health outcomes across a wide range of health care interventions. Thus, it is of particular interest to demonstrate the extent to which DCEs can fulfil a generalizable role for health care priority setting and resource allocation decisions. Although information on this issue is currently lacking (Dowie 1998), a future research direction would be to build on the *benefit transfer* literature published by environmental economists (e.g. Morrison *et al.* 2002). Benefit transfer relates to the notion of assessing whether DCE models can be transferred or adapted to construct valuations for resources that are different in type, location or time, from the one originally studied (Smith 1993).

CONCLUSIONS

This chapter has discussed the role of the DCE technique in producing valid and versatile measures of benefit in health economics, particularly for health economic evaluation but also for other uses. It is expected that DCEs will be used more. However, a number of key methodological concerns remain. Some of these have been highlighted and serve as a useful agenda for future research in this area. These relate to: having a better understanding of how respondents interpret price and risk attributes; comparing direct willingness to pay and DCEs in empirical studies; understanding the most appropriate way to ask the question; strengthening analysis; investigating decision-making heuristics employed when completing DCEs and the extent to which these are related to the complexity of the task; external validity; the impact of strategic behaviour; face validity; and generalizability. Collaborative work with design experts, psychologists, sociologists and qualitative researchers should prove useful when investigating these issues. It is clearly also necessary to link this research agenda to work being carried out in marketing, transport economics and environmental economics, and health economics benefit assessment more generally.

ACKNOWLEDGEMENTS

The authors would like to thank Emma McIntosh and participants of the HERU workshop for comments on earlier drafts. Funding is acknowledged from the Medical Research Council, South East NHS Executive and the Chief Scientist Office of the Scottish Executive Health Department. The views, however, are those of the authors.

REFERENCES

Adamowicz W (2001) Personal communication, International Health Economic Conference, University of York.

Blumenschein K, Johannesson M, Yokoyama K and Freeman P (2001) Hypothetical versus real willingness to pay in the health care sector. *Journal of Health Economics*, **20**, 441–457.

Cairns J and van der Pol M (2000) The estimation of marginal time preference in a UK-wide sample (TEMPUS) project. *Health Technology Assessment*, **4**(1).

Carlsson F and Martinnsson P (2002) Do hypothetical and actual marginal willingness to pay differ in choice experiments? *Journal of Environmental Economics and Management*, **41**, 179–192.

Chakraborty G, Ettensen R and Gaeth G (1994) How consumers choose health insurance. *Journal of Health Care Marketing*, **14**, 21–33.

Clark P (2002) Testing the convergent validity of the contingent valuation and travel cost methods in valuing the benefits of health care. *Health Economics*, **11**, 117–127.

Department of the Environment, Transport and the Regions' Highways (1997) Economics Note 2, November 1997. In *Design Manuals for Roads and Bridges, Volume 13*. TSO, London.

De Palma A, Myers G and Papageorgious Y (1994) Rational choice under an imperfect ability to choose. *American Economic Review*, **84**, 419–440.

Dowie J (1998) *Process utility, conjoint analysis and willingness to pay*. Paper presented to the Health Economic Study Group Meeting, University of Galway.

Farrar S, Ryan M, Ross D and Ludbrook A (2000) Using discrete choice modelling in priority setting: an application to clinical service developments. *Social Science and Medicine*, **50**, 63–75.

Fischer G and Hawkins S (1993) Strategy compatibility, scale compatibility and the prominence effect. *Journal of Experimental Psychology: Human Perception and Performance*, **19**, 580–597.

Gerard K (2002) *Respondent consistency in discrete choice experiments: moving things forward using a case study in emergency and on demand health care systems*. Paper presented at the Discrete Choice Workshop, University of Southern Denmark, Odense.

Gigerenzer G and Todd P for the ABC Research Group (1999) *Simple Heuristics that Make us Smart*. Oxford University Press, New York.

Godsen T, Bowler I and Sutton M (2000) How do general practitioners choose their practice? Preferences for practice and job characteristics. *Journal of Health Services Research and Policy*, 5(4), 208–213.

Hakim Z and Pathak D (1999) Modeling the EuroQol data: A comparison of discrete choice conjoint and conditional preference modelling. *Health Economics*, **8**, 103–116.

Hanemann W (1984) Welfare evaluations in contingent valuation experiments with discrete responses: Reply. *American Journal of Agricultural Economics*, **69**, 332–341.

Hanley N, Mourato S and Wright R (2001) Choice modelling: a superior alternative for environmental valuation? *Journal of Economic Surveys*, **15**, 435–462.

Heiner R (1983) The origin of predictable behaviour. *American Economic Review*, **73**, 560–595.

Hensher D, Stopher P and Louviere J (2001) An exploratory analysis of the effect of numbers of choices sets in designed choice experiments: an airline choice application. *Journal of Air Transport Management*, **2**, 373–370.

Huber J and Zwerina K (1996) The importance of utility balance in efficient choice designs. *Journal of Marketing Research*, **33**, 307–317.

Jan S, Mooney G, Ryan M, Bruggeman K and Alexander K (2000) The use of conjoint analysis to elicit community preferences in public health research: a case study of hospital services in Australia. *Australian and New Zealand Journal of Public Health*, **24**(1), 64–70.

Johnson R, Banzhaf M and Desvousges W (2000) Willingness to pay for improved respiratory and cardiovascular health: a multiple-format, stated preference approach. *Health Economics*, **9**, 295–317.

Kahneman D, Slovic P and Tversky A (1982) *Judgement under Uncertainty: Heuristics and Biases*. Cambridge University Press, Cambridge.

Lancaster K (1966) A new approach to consumer theory. *Journal of Political Economy*, **74**, 134–157.

Lancaster K (1971) *Consumer Demand*. Columbia University Press, New York.

Lattimer V, Brailsford S, Gerard K, George S, Smith H, Turnbull T, Tarnaras P and Maslin-Prothero S (2002) *Nottingham Emergency Care/On Demand Services Project*. Research Project, University of Southampton.

Lloyd A (2001) The extent of patients' understanding of the risk of treatments. *Quality in Health Care*, **10**(suppl. I), i14–i18.

Loomes G and Sugden R (1992) Regret theory: an alternative theory of rational choice under uncertainty. *Economic Journal*, **92**, 805–824.

Louviere J, Oppewal H, Timmermans H and Thomas T (1997) *Handling large numbers of attributes in conjoint applications: Who says existing techniques can't be applied? But if you want an alternative, how about hierarchical choice experiments?* Mimeograph.

Luce RD (1959) *Individual Choice Behaviour: a Theoretical Analysis*. Wiley, New York.

McFadden D (1973) *Conditional logit analysis of qualitative choice behaviour*. University of California at Berkeley, California.

McIntosh E and Ryan M (2002) Discrete choice experiments to derive welfare estimates for the provision of elective surgery: implications of discontinuous preferences. *Journal of Economic Psychology*, **23**(3), 367–382.

Morrison M, Bennett J, Blamey R and Louviere J (2002) Choice modelling and tests of benefit transfer. *Journal of Agricultural Economics*, **84**(1), 161–170.

Netten A, Ryan M, Skåtun D and Smith P (2000) *Establishing preferences of older people for domains of outcome of social care*. Paper presented to British Society of Gerontology, University of York.

Ohler T, Le A, Louviere J and Swait J (2000) Attribute range effects in binary response tasks. *Marketing Letters*, **11**, 249–260.

Payne J, Bettman J and Johnson E (1993) *The Adaptive Decision-maker*. Cambridge University Press, New York.

Pearmain D, Swanson J, Kroes E and Bradley M (1991) *Stated Preference Techniques: a Guide to Practice*. Steer Davis Gleave and Hague Consulting Group, Hague.

Ratcliffe J and Longworth L (2002) Investigating structural reliability within health technology assessment: a discrete choice experiment. *International Journal of Technology Assessment*, **18**(1), 139–144.

Revelt D and Train K (1998) Mixed logit with repeated choices: Households' choices of appliance efficiency level. *Review of Economics and Statistics*, **80**, 647–657.

Ryan M and Gerard K (2001) *Using choice experiments to value health care programmes: current practice and future challenges*. Paper presented at International Health Economic Association Conference, University of York.

Ryan M and San Miguel F (2002) Revisiting the axiom of completeness in health care. *Health Economics* (forthcoming).

Ryan M and Wordsworth S (2000) Sensitivity of willingness to pay estimates to the level of attributes in discrete choice experiments. *Scottish Journal of Political Economy*, **47**(5), 504–524.

Ryan M, Scott DA, Reeves C, Bate A, van Teijlingen E, Russell E, Napper M and Robb C (2001a) Eliciting public preferences for health care: a systematic review of techniques. *Health Technology Assessment*, **5**(5).

Ryan M, Bate A, Eastmond C and Ludbrook A (2001b) Using discrete choice experiments to elicit preferences. *Quality in Health Care*, **10**, 155–160.

Ryan M, Reeves C and Entwistle V (2002) *Listening to respondents: a think aloud study of Discrete Choice Experiment responses*. Paper presented to the Health Economic Study Group Meeting, University of East Anglia.

San Miguel F (2002) *Testing the assumptions of completeness, stability and rationality of preferences using discrete choice experiments*. PhD Thesis, University of Aberdeen.

Schkade D and Payne J (1994) How people respond to contingent valuation questions: A verbal protocol analysis of willingness to pay for an environmental regulation. *Journal of Environmental Economics and Management*, **26**, 88–109.

Scott A (2000) Eliciting GPs' preferences for pecuniary and non-pecuniary job characteristics. *Journal of Health Economics*, **711**, 1–19.

Simon H (1955) Behavioural model of rational choice. *Quarterly Journal of Economics*, **69**, 99–118.

Smith V (1993) Non-market valuation of environmental resources: an interpretative appraisal. *Land Economy*, **69**, 1–26.

Strensund J, Sylvestre E and Sivadas E (1997) Targeting Medicare consumers. *Marketing Health Services*, **2**, 8–17.

Swait J (2001) A non-compensatory choice model incorporating attribute cut-offs. *Transportation Research*, **35**, 903–928.

Szeinbach SL, Barnes JH, McGhan WF, Murawski MM and Corey R (1999) Using conjoint analysis to evaluate health state preferences. *Drug Information Journal*, **33**, 849–858.

van der Pol M and Cairns J (1998) Establishing patient preferences for blood transfusion support: an application of conjoint analysis. *Journal of Health Services Research and Policy*, 3(2), 70–76.

Vick S and Scott A (1998) Agency in health care. Examining patients' preferences for attributes of the doctor–patient relationship. *Journal of Health Economics*, **17**(5), 587–605.

3

Methods for Eliciting Time Preferences Over Future Health Events

MARJON VAN DER POL
Department of Community Health Sciences & Centre for Health and Policy Studies,
University of Calgary

JOHN CAIRNS
Health Economics Research Unit, University of Aberdeen

INTRODUCTION

There is a growing literature on the elicitation of intertemporal preferences over future health events. The aim of this chapter is to provide an overview of the methods used to elicit these preferences, to highlight the differences between the methods and to identify outstanding research questions. A taxonomy of the methods that have been used to elicit time preferences for health events is first presented, followed by detailed examples of the approaches to eliciting time preferences. The main differences between the methods and their advantages and disadvantages are then described. The chapter closes with a discussion of the outstanding research questions in this area.

Interest in how individuals regard future health events has two main sources: a concern over the appropriate methods for taking timing into account in economic evaluations; and a desire to obtain a better understanding of individual health-affecting behaviour. Discounting practices often play a central role in determining the relative cost-effectiveness of different interventions. There is an ongoing debate concerning the choice of social discount rate for use in the evaluation of health care. Current practice (in most countries) is that future health benefits are discounted at the same rate as future monetary

Advances in Health Economics. Edited by Anthony Scott, Alan Maynard and Robert Elliott.
© 2003 John Wiley & Sons, Ltd

costs. One normative view is that consumer sovereignty should form the basis for discounting in economic evaluation and therefore the rate that best represents people's preferences should be used to discount future health benefits.

Another reason for the interest in time preferences for health is a desire to obtain a better understanding of individual health-affecting behaviour. One of the factors influencing health-affecting behaviour, like smoking and exercising, is likely to be intertemporal preferences. Lifestyle choices generally involve a trade-off between current costs and future benefits. For example, giving up smoking involves costs now in terms of foregone pleasure and the experience of withdrawal symptoms and future benefits, such as improved quality of life and increased life expectancy. Because these lifestyle choices involve trade-offs between current costs and future benefits, intertemporal preferences are likely to influence whether individuals give up smoking, whether they exercise, etc.

Several research questions are generated by the twin concerns of understanding health-affecting behaviour and informing discounting practice. One important research question is whether individual private time preferences for health are similar to their social time preferences. Another is whether time preferences for health are domain-independent, that is, do individuals discount different health outcomes at the same rate. At first sight the existence of long-run differences in implied rates for different outcomes might seem strange, in that elsewhere in the economy pressures are expected to equalize rates of return on different assets. However, in the case of individual health the scope for such arbitrage is limited. Another part of the research agenda is whether the underlying model, the discounted utility model, accurately describes individuals' time preferences for health. Finally, there is a need to research the relationship between individuals' time preferences for health and health-affecting behaviour. The choice of method to elicit time preferences may in some cases depend on the research question that is to be addressed.

It is necessary to consider more closely what is meant by time preference, particularly since authors differ with respect to what they refer to as time preference. Related to this discussion are questions regarding whether or not, in principle, time preferences for health events are measurable. In a paper predating all of the empirical work by about five years, Gafni and Torrance (1984) identified three distinct effects which make up an individual's attitude to risk in a health context: a quantity effect; a time preference effect; and a gambling effect. The time preference effect is sometimes described as *pure* time preference (or somewhat pejoratively as impatience). Other authors (for example, Olson & Bailey 1981) would argue that diminishing marginal utility (the quantity effect) and the risk attached to any future event are also elements of time preference.

Before anyone had attempted to measure time preferences for health events, Gafni and Torrance (1984) expressed some early optimism. They suggested that time preference could be 'measured by asking conventional time preference questions ... but cast in the health, as opposed to financial domain' and claimed that it was not necessary to speculate on the nature of time preference '... since it is empirically determinable' (p. 449). However, drawing on Loewenstein and Prelec (1993), which highlighted the importance of another class of effects that affect intertemporal choice – sequence effects, Gafni (1995) argues robustly that no measurement technique allows pure time preference to be distinguished. The best that can be achieved is a measure of time preference for a given sequence of events. This may be true of preferences over one's own future health states. However, it is less clear that the sequence of events will be an important influence when considering preferences over life-saving profiles. In any case, Gyrd-Hansen and Søgaard (1998) argue that for economic evaluation we do not require a measure of pure time preferences but that we also wish to include diminishing marginal utility and uncertainty. From this perspective, it is an advantage if more than pure time preferences are captured by the elicitation method.

Given these conceptual issues and also the special nature of the commodity health there are clearly many challenges to be faced when eliciting these preferences. Researchers have responded to these challenges by adopting a wide range of methods in their empirical work, and these are described in the next section.

TAXONOMY OF METHODS FOR ELICITING TIME PREFERENCES

Two broad approaches have been used to estimate time preference rates – revealed preference and stated preference. The distinction is that the former involves observing actual behaviour whereas the latter involves asking individuals what they would do in particular *hypothetical* circumstances. Revealed preference methods for estimating time preference can be divided into three categories (Fredericks *et al.* 2002). The first category derives time preference rates from behaviours that involve trade-offs between outcomes over time, such as the purchase of consumer durables (Hausman 1979) and educational investment decisions (Lang & Ruud 1986). Time preference rates can also be estimated by observing how individuals trade off wage and risk, which can be interpreted as a trade-off between quality of life and life expectancy (Viscusi & Moore 1989). A third category derives time preference rates through the estimation of structural models of lifecycle saving behaviour. It should be noted that this method cannot be applied to derive a rate for health outcomes.

Economists generally prefer revealed preference methods to stated preference methods. However, in health economics there is a recognition that the special nature of health and health care results in there being many fewer opportunities to obtain valuations from observed behaviour. This is especially so in the case of time preferences for health. Individuals could invest in their future health by adopting a healthy lifestyle now, or they could invest in health insurance, but these opportunities to trade are limited, especially compared to the opportunities to trade wealth across time. Another limitation of using revealed preference methods is that the estimation of time preference rates is relatively indirect and quite complicated. This results partly from the difficulty of using data collected primarily for some other purpose and the many more factors outwith the researcher's control (as compared with an experimental approach). There are often many confounding factors present. Because the scope for using revealed preferences to derive time preferences for health is limited, and because the methods used are more specific to individual studies, the remainder of this chapter focuses on stated preference methods.

The stated preference methods can be classified as open-ended (or matching) methods, closed-ended (or choice) methods, or rating/pricing methods. Matching studies have been undertaken as fully open-ended or using the time preference equivalent of a payment card. Four different approaches have been adopted to estimate time preference using choice or closed-ended questions: discrete choice; discrete choice with follow-up; discrete choice with repeated follow-up; and discrete choice experiments. Rating methods elicit a score for a temporal prospect, for example, a health profile. An implied time preference rate is estimated by comparing scores for different temporal prospects. Pricing methods are similar to rating methods but elicit willingness to pay for temporal prospects instead of a score. Rating and pricing methods differ from the open-ended and closed-ended methods in that they do not present individuals directly with trade-offs between outcomes at different points in time.

When using stated preference approaches to elicit time preferences for health there are numerous potential differences in design between studies in terms of the way in which the questions are framed. For example, in the case of non-fatal changes in health state with respect to: base health state; number of different health states; time horizon; and whether or not the comparison is between points in time or profiles. The base health state can be full-health and subjects make choices with respect to the consumption of ill-health (Redelmeier & Heller 1993) or the base health state is ill-health and subjects make choices with respect to the consumption of full-health (Chapman & Elstein 1995). Some studies consider only one ill-health state (Cairns 1992), others have considered more than one ill-health state (Dolan & Gudex 1995). A limited time period can be considered (Chapman 1996) (for instance five years), or a scenario can describe remaining life (Enemark *et al.* 1998). Subjects can be asked to consider two points in time or they can be presented with a profile.

The standard approach has been the former, with few studies comparing profiles (Chapman *et al*. 1999).

In principle, studies asking matching questions could ask subjects to specify: the *timing* of a given change in health; or the *magnitude* to be experienced at a certain point of time; or possibly the health-related *quality of life* to be experienced. However, no study has asked individuals to specify timing or quality of life. Studies have asked individuals to specify the magnitude of a specified health benefit to be enjoyed at a particular point in the future either in terms of: lives saved (Olsen 1993); or duration of health state (Cairns & van der Pol 2000); or frequency of symptoms (Chapman *et al*. 1999).

EXAMPLES OF STATED PREFERENCE METHODS

In order to facilitate comparison of the different methods and to simplify the exposition, the detailed examples of the different elicitation methods are presented holding a number of factors constant throughout. Private preferences are elicited for non-fatal changes in health framed in terms of losses, specifically, durations of ill-health. To keep the questions relatively simple only one health state and one spell of ill-health are considered. The spell of ill-health occurs at two points in time only, namely s and v. Preferences are elicited under conditions of certainty. Each example shows the type of intertemporal question associated with the elicitation method and demonstrates the method of analysis. See Tables 3.1 and 3.2 for references to applications of the different methods.

FRAMEWORK

Time preferences are generally measured assuming the discounted utility (DU) model. In the DU model time preferences are captured by a single time preference rate denoted as ρ. The intertemporal utility function can be expressed as:

$$V(x_1, x_2, \ldots, x_t) = \sum_{t=1}^{T} \left(\frac{1}{1+\rho}\right)^t v(x_t)$$

where x_t is the duration of ill-health occurring at time t.

OPEN-ENDED/MATCHING

The time preference rate is estimated by identifying an indifference point between two durations of ill-health which occur at two different points in time. These outcomes are denoted by x_s and x'_v where $s < v$. In an open-ended question the subject is asked to return a value thereby eliciting an indifference point

Table 3.1 Studies of time preferences for health states

	Method	Sample
Open-ended		
Cairns (1992)	Fully open-ended	29 students
Olsen (1993)	Fully open-ended	250 general public &
		77 planners
Chapman & Elstein (1995)	Fully open-ended	104 students
Chapman (1996)	Fully open-ended	148 students
Cairns & van der Pol (1999)	Payment scale	298 general public
Chapman & Coups (1999)	Payment scale	409 employees
Lazaro et al. (2001)	Payment scale	203 students
Lazaro et al. (2002)	Payment scale	427 general public
Closed-ended		
Chapman et al. (1999)	DC repeated follow-up	79 patients & 77 students
van der Pol & Cairns (1999)	DC with follow-up	367 general public
Ganiats et al. (2000)	Single DC	169 patients
Bleichrodt & Johannesson	DC experiment	172 students
(2001)		
Cairns & van der Pol (2001)	DC repeated follow-up	203 students
van der Pol & Cairns (2001)	DC experiment	158 general public
Rating/pricing		
Lipscomb (1989)	VAS	52 students
MacKeigan et al. (1993)	VAS	108 students & hospital
		volunteers
Redelmeier & Heller (1993)	SG & VAS	121 students & doctors
Olsen (1994)	TTO	90 students & 40 doctors
Dolan & Gudex (1995)	TTO	39 general public
Stavem et al. (2002)	TTO	59 patients

$(x_s \sim x'_v)$. A choice has to be made as to which value the subject is asked to return. In the example the subject is given values for v, s and x, and returns a value for x':

Scenario A: you are ill for 30 days in 2 years' time
Scenario B: you are ill for ____ days in 4 years' time

To make the question slightly easier to answer a visual aid containing a range of possible responses can be provided to subjects. This method is referred to as the payment card technique in the area of contingent valuation. Since each question elicits an indifference point the estimation of the time preference rate is straightforward. Assuming the DU model the time preference rate is equal to:

Table 3.2 Studies of time preferences for lives and life years

	Method	Sample
Open-ended		
Olsen (1993)	Fully open-ended	250 general public & 77 planners
Cairns (1994)	Payment scale	223 general public
Cairns & van der Pol (1997a,b)	Payment scale	473 general public
Enemark *et al.* (1998)	SG	25 surgeons
Lazaro *et al.* (2001)	Payment scale	203 students
Gyrd-Hansen (2002)	Fully open-ended & SG	79 students
Höjgård *et al.* (2002)	SG	66 doctors, 21 patients, 22 general public
Lazaro *et al.* (2002)	Payment scale	427 general public
Closed-ended		
Horowitz & Carson (1990)	Single DC	75 students
Cropper *et al.* (1991)	DC with follow-up	1600 general public
Cropper *et al.* (1994)	DC with follow-up	3200 general public
Johannesson & Johansson (1996)	Single DC	850 general public
Ganiats *et al.* (2000)	Single DC	169 patients
Poulos & Whittington (2000)	Single DC	3127 general public
Rating/pricing		
Johannesson & Johansson (1997a)	WTP	528 general public
Johannesson & Johansson (1997b)	WTP	2577 general public
Gyrd-Hansen (2002)	TTO, PTO	79 students

$$\rho = (x'_v/x_s)^{1/(v-s)} - 1$$

An alternative open-ended method which introduces uncertainty is the use of a standard gamble (SG) to elicit time preferences. For example, subjects can be presented with a choice between living another 20 years or taking medication which would result in a probability p of living another 40 years and a probability $(1-p)$ of living another 10 years. Once a value for p is returned the implied time preference rate can be obtained by solving the following equation:

$$\frac{(1+\rho)^{20}-1}{(1+\rho)^{20} \times \rho} = \frac{(1+\rho)^{40}-1}{(1+\rho)^{40} \times \rho} \times p + \frac{(1+\rho)^{10}-1}{(1+\rho)^{10} \times \rho} \times (1-p)$$

CLOSED-ENDED/CHOICE

When using a closed-ended method all values for x, x', s and v are specified and the subject is asked to indicate which scenario s/he prefers. This kind of question is also called a dichotomous choice, a pairwise comparison and a discrete choice. An example of a discrete choice is:

Which scenario is least bad?
☐ Scenario A: you are ill for 30 days in 2 years' time
☒ Scenario B: you are ill for 39 days in 4 years' time
☐ Scenario A and B are equally bad

Assuming the DU model each discrete choice implies a discount rate denoted as r:

$$r = (x'_v/x_s)^{1/(v-s)} - 1$$

Indifference between scenario A and B implies that the individual's time preference rate is equal to the discount rate offered in the discrete choice. If an individual prefers scenario B, his/her time preference rate is higher than the discount rate offered in the choice and similarly if the individual prefers scenario A, his/her time preference rate is lower than the rate offered.

There are several closed-ended methods which differ mainly in terms of how many choices the subject is presented with. Four different methods are described here: single discrete choice; discrete choice with follow-up; discrete choice with repeated follow-up; and discrete choice experiment.

Single Discrete Choice

This method presents subjects with one single discrete choice only. The population's underlying distribution of time preferences is identified by randomly assigning discrete choices implying a number of different discount rates, also called the bid vector. The appropriate bid vector can be determined using methods based on prior information on the underlying distribution (see for example Cooper 1993). Since only limited information is available for each subject a time preference rate can only be estimated for the whole sample. Regression analysis is used to model individuals' preferences as a function of the discount rate offered in the choice and individuals' characteristics. The mean rate is then estimated using the regression coefficients (see Cameron 1988 for details).

Discrete Choice with Follow-up

To increase statistical efficiency a follow-up choice can be introduced. The discount rate offered in the follow-up choice depends on the answer to the initial choice. If an individual prefers scenario A the follow-up choice will imply a lower discount rate. If an individual prefers scenario B the follow-up choice will imply a higher discount rate. The implied time preference rate can be varied by manipulating either the value for x, x', s or v. The estimation of the mean time preference rate is the same as for the single discrete choice apart from the use of a regression model which allows for the double-bounded nature of the data (see Cameron & Quiggin 1994).

Discrete Choice with Repeated Follow-up

This method is an extended version of the discrete choice with follow-up. Subjects are presented with additional follow-up choices until an indifference point is identified. This is done using an iterative method in which the discount rate offered in the follow-up choice is contingent upon the answer to the previous choice. A substantial number of choices may be required to identify the subject's indifference point and it may therefore be more feasible to stop the exercise once the subject's responses indicate a time preference rate within a pre-specified interval. Since an indifference point is identified for each individual the estimation of the implied time preference rate is the same as for the open-ended method. Some subjects may have lexicographic preferences, that is, they prefer scenario A (B) independent of the duration of ill-health in scenario B. For these subjects a time preference rate cannot be estimated.

Discrete Choice Experiment

In a discrete choice experiment subjects are presented with several discrete choices which imply a range of discount rates. This method is similar to the single discrete choice with the main difference that each subject is presented with all of the 'bids'. There are several ways in which the data can be analysed. One way is to extend the model used for the single discrete choice. A more common way is to model the utility differences between the two scenarios. In the case of time preferences there is a difference in terms of durations of ill-health and when they occur:

$$U_B - U_A = \alpha + \beta_1(x_{2B} - x_{2A}) + \beta_2(x_{4B} - x_{4A}) + \varepsilon$$

where x_{tA} is the duration of ill-health at time t in scenario A and x_{tB} is the duration of ill-health occurring at time t in scenario B. Assuming the DU model, the implied time preference rate for the 2-year delay is:

$$\rho = (\beta_1/\beta_2)^{1/2} - 1$$

RATING/PRICING METHODS

Instead of presenting individuals directly with trade-offs between periods of ill-health over time, time preferences can be elicited by obtaining utility scores for different health profiles. These profiles differ in terms of when the ill-health occurs. The utility scores can be elicited using a visual analogue scale (VAS) or time trade-off (TTO). A rating scale example is:

On a scale from 0 to 10 rank the following two profiles:
1. You are ill for 30 days in 2 years' time   _____
2. You are ill for 30 days in 4 years' time   _____

The implied time preference rate is equal to:

$$\rho = (U_{x'_v}/U_{x_s})^{1/(v-s)} - 1$$

where U_{xt} is the utility score for x days of ill-health at time t.

When using pricing methods a willingness to pay value is elicited for different health profiles. An example is:

How much are you willing to pay to avoid:
1. Being ill for 30 days in 2 years' time   _____
2. Being ill for 30 days in 4 years' time   _____

The implied time preference rate is equal to:

$$\rho = (WTP_{x'_v}/WTP_{x_s})^{1/(v-s)} - 1$$

where WTP_{xt} is the willingness to pay to avoid x days of ill-health at time t.

This section has outlined a range of approaches that can be, and in some form have been, used to elicit time preferences with respect to future health events. In order to facilitate the comparison several factors have been held constant. This masks various choices that the researcher has to make, for example, with respect to the health state, the period of delay, the range and intervals to use (in the case of a payment scale), etc. The examples used non-fatal changes in health but similar approaches can be used to elicit time preferences for statistical lives saved. For example, an individual can be presented with a trade-off between saving 1000 lives one year from now and 1500 lives seven years from now.

In order to demonstrate the extent to which these different approaches have been applied in practice, Tables 3.1 and 3.2 summarize the empirical work on time preferences with respect to health states and lives and life years respectively. The studies have been grouped into those using open-ended methods, those using closed-ended methods, and those using rating/pricing methods to elicit time preferences. The tables show the method and the sample used. Several different methods have been applied. There appears to be no preference for a particular method in that open-ended, closed-ended and rating/pricing methods have been applied to roughly the same extent. Closed-ended methods have only been employed in recent years with respect to health states, whereas closed-ended methods have been overtaken in popularity by open-ended methods in the case of lives or life-years saved.

CRITERIA FOR CHOOSING BETWEEN METHODS

The primary concern is with the validity of the time preferences elicited by a particular method, that is, do the estimated preferences represent the individual's true preferences. Evidence of validity can take a number of forms, for example, close agreement between stated preference and revealed preference methods, and differences in observed behaviour being predicted by differences in estimated time preferences. There is, however, relatively little evidence available on the validity or otherwise of the different preference elicitation methods.

VALIDITY

In the absence of data on revealed preferences, the convergent validity of different stated preference approaches might be considered, although different methods giving similar results does not guarantee that they are accurate representations of individuals' preferences. While different methods have been used before, it is difficult to compare the estimated rates of time preference because of the many differences between the studies. For instance, there is substantial evidence that implied discount rates are a function of the period of delay (Cairns & van der Pol 1997b). It is therefore difficult to compare studies which offer different periods of delay. There have been only two studies that were designed to directly compare estimates of time preferences across methods. Cairns and van der Pol (2000) compared an open-ended method with a discrete choice experiment. The mean rates were higher in case of the open-ended questions but most of the differences were neither statistically significant nor large. Gyrd-Hansen (2002) compared an SG method and a rating method (TTO). The SG elicited higher rates than the TTO method.

There is substantial evidence in areas other than time preferences for health that different elicitation methods produce different results. It has been shown in the psychology literature that preference reversal occurs when switching from a closed-ended to an open-ended method. This has been tested mainly in the context of monetary gambles and it is unclear whether the result can be generalized into the health domain. There is also substantial evidence in the area of contingent valuation that different methods produce different mean willingness to pay values (see for example Brown *et al.* 1996). These differences in results have often been explained in terms of differences in how individuals perceive the question, in particular, in terms of differences in incentives for individuals to act strategically (Carson 1997). In the case of time preferences for health there do not seem to be any obvious incentives to respond strategically in any of the elicitation methods, and it can therefore not be assumed that the findings in the contingent valuation literature apply to time preferences. The differences in contingent valuation studies have also been explained in terms of estimation bias. For instance, Halvorsen and Sælensminde (1998) found that violation of the homoscedasticity assumption leads to biased WTP estimates if the error terms are correlated with the costs.

Successful prediction of the determinants of individual time preference rates might also be taken as evidence of the validity of the method. The individual characteristic most commonly found to be significantly associated with the implied time preference rate is the age of the subject. As might be anticipated, older subjects tend to have higher time preference rates. There is limited evidence of significant associations between implied time preference rates and a number of other variables, including presence of young children in the household, ethnic group, smoking status and gender.

Since choice of method cannot currently be based solely on evidence of validity, other characteristics, or advantages and disadvantages, of the different methods become of increased importance. The main potential differences between the methods are in terms of statistical efficiency, richness of the data, cognitive difficulty, strategic behaviour and potential biases.

STATISTICAL EFFICIENCY

Closed-ended methods are generally less efficient than open-ended and rating/ pricing methods (Carson 2000). In particular, the single discrete choice is statistically inefficient in that large sample sizes are required to identify the underlying distribution of time preferences with any given degree of accuracy. Statistical efficiency is improved by introducing one or more follow-up questions or by using a discrete choice experiment. The difference in statistical efficiency across methods becomes important when the sample size available to researchers is considerably restricted, for example, by resources available to conduct the research. In these circumstances eliciting time preferences using, for instance, a single discrete choice is unlikely to be feasible.

RICHNESS OF DATA

Open-ended and rating/pricing methods generally produce a richer data set in that individual-level data are obtained. Using these methods implied time preference rates are identifiable for individual subjects and not just for the group. Time preference rates can only be estimated for the group when using closed-ended methods, with the exception of the discrete choice with repeated follow-up. For some purposes individual-level data are essential, for example, when comparing different time preference functions individual-level data are required to enable the modelling of the alternative functions.

COGNITIVE DIFFICULTY

The psychology literature shows that closed-ended questions are generally easier to answer than open-ended questions (Tversky *et al.* 1988). To answer open-ended questions subjects have to make quantitative comparisons. Rather than expressing a preference they have to return a specific value that represents their preferences. It should be noted that discrete choices may still require considerable cognitive effort in the case of time preferences. Intertemporal questions are complex by nature. Thinking about the future is not easy, especially in the context of health. Subjects are also unlikely to be familiar with these kind of questions. It could be argued that the rating/pricing methods are cognitively less demanding since the subject does not have to directly trade off two different health outcomes at two different points in time.

It should also be noted that although discrete choices may be easier to answer, the cognitive effort required will increase as the number of choices the subject is presented with increase. So a discrete choice experiment may be as demanding as a single open-ended question. The implication of the differences in cognitive difficulty is that if the cognitive skills of the study sample are limited to some extent some questions may be less appropriate. For example, it may be more appropriate to use a single discrete choice to elicit preferences when using a random sample of the general public, since it is unknown whether this sample will have the cognitive skills required. The cognitive difficulty of the questions is clearly likely to influence the response rate.

STRATEGIES

Another way in which methods may differ is in terms of the strategies subjects use to answer the questions. Payne *et al.* (1993) argued that preferences are constructed during the elicitation process and that individuals develop strategies that enable them to minimize effort while preserving accuracy. These strategies or heuristics vary across elicitation methods. Tversky *et al.* (1988) described one way in which they might differ. They hypothesized that the more prominent attribute weighs more heavily in choice than in open-ended questions. When using choices to elicit preferences individuals decide according to the more prominent attribute, say duration of ill-health. The open-ended question cannot be resolved in the same manner. Attributes are likely to be weighted more equally in an open-ended question.

POTENTIAL BIASES

The potential biases differ across the elicitation methods. A potential bias when using more than one discrete choice to elicit preferences is an anchoring effect or starting point bias. This means that the first choice influences subsequent choices. There is also a potential estimation bias when using closed-ended questions. Generally, strong assumptions of the form and distribution of the underlying utility function are required to obtain estimates of the time preference rate (unless an indifference point is elicited for each individual). Violations of these assumptions may lead to biased estimates.

Framing effects are likely to be present when using an open-ended method since a choice needs to be made as to which value the subject has to return. For example, the health outcome can either be delayed or expedited. Evidence suggests that the time preference rate is higher when the health outcome is delayed (Cairns 1992).

A potential bias when using rating/pricing methods or standard gamble is that the DU model has to be assumed in order to estimate the time preference rate. Evidence suggests that this model does not accurately describe individuals' preferences (Cairns & van der Pol 1997a,b).

Since there is currently only limited evidence on the validity of the different methods, the choice of method is most likely to be made by weighing the relative advantages and disadvantages. Table 3.3 is an attempt to summarize the relative (dis)advantages. It should be noted that these are broad-brush characterizations, and that a particular method might reasonably be scored differently depending on the specific context. Also, importantly, the weight attached to the different criteria will depend on the particular aims of the study. While the extent of potential bias will always be an important consideration, ease of answering will be more important when the aim is to produce representative estimates of time preferences. The weight attached to the size of sample a method requires will vary depending on the resource constraints facing the researcher.

The summary shows that there is neither a superior nor an inferior method. When using open-ended questions or the discrete choice with repeated follow-up there is a trade-off between richness of information and sample size and

Table 3.3 Summary of relative (dis)advantages

Method	Small sample	Richness of data	Easy to answer	Unbiased estimates
Open-ended	+ +	+ +	− −	+ −
DC	− −	− −	+ +	+ +
DC with follow-up	−	−	+	+
DC repeated follow-up	+ +	+ +	+ −	−
DC experiment	+	+ −	+ −	+
Rating/pricing	+ +	+	+	− −

cognitive difficulty and biased estimates. The opposite holds for the single discrete choice with or without follow-up. The rating/pricing method scores quite well on most factors but is also most likely to produce biased estimates.

RESEARCH QUESTIONS

This chapter has identified the range of methods that have been used to elicit time preferences over future health events. Several research questions concerning these elicitation methods can be identified. One question is whether there are any new approaches that could be explored. Most of the methods described in this chapter are closely related to the methods used in the area of contingent valuation. Can any other contingent valuation methods be adapted for use with respect to time preferences, or are there any other suitable methods which have not formed part of the contingent valuation research programme?

This chapter has shown that in the context of these time preferences there is only very limited evidence available on the validity of the different stated preference methods. This lack of evidence should be addressed by future research. The first step is to examine the influence of different methods of eliciting preferences on estimates of time preference rates. One interesting way of testing this would be to replicate the experiments used in the psychology literature designed to test for preference reversal. This would also provide the opportunity to examine subjects' decision-making when answering time preference questions and whether they use particular strategies.

The available empirical evidence has shown that time preference rates vary widely across individuals, across studies and vary across health outcomes. The wide variation in estimated time preference rates could raise concern regarding the validity of the stated preference methods used. Time preference questions are complex. Part of the problem is that most individuals are simply unused to thinking in the way required of them. Consumers make many different choices with intertemporal implications but these implications, while not certain, are perhaps characterized by less uncertainty than intertemporal health choices. A related difficulty is that of devising questions which are meaningful to the individual. Thus there are always likely to be doubts about the extent to which these methods have enabled researchers to accurately elicit time preferences. This raises the question whether research efforts should focus on refining the stated preference methods. It may be more fruitful to shift the emphasis towards obtaining corroboration of findings using revealed preference methods. Examining the relationship between implied time preferences and differences in behaviour is an important step in that direction. The paucity to date of studies of this kind belies the enormous potential for such research.

ACKNOWLEDGEMENTS

The authors would like to thank John Hutton and others who attended the HERU workshop for useful comments on an earlier draft. HERU is funded by the Chief Scientist Office of the Scottish Executive Health Department. The views in this chapter are those of the authors.

REFERENCES

Bleichrodt H and Johannesson M (2001) An empirical test of stationarity versus generalized stationarity. *Journal of Mathematical Psychology*, **45**, 265–282.
Brown TC, Champ PA, Bishop RC and McCollum DW (1996) Which response format reveals the truth about donations to a public good. *Land Economics*, **72**, 152–166.
Cairns JA (1992) Health, wealth and time preference. *Project Appraisal*, **7**, 31–40.
Cairns JA (1994) Valuing future benefits. *Health Economics*, **3**, 221–229.
Cairns JA and van der Pol MM (1997a) Saving future lives: a comparison of three discounting models. *Health Economics*, **6**, 341–350.
Cairns JA and van der Pol MM (1997b) Constant and decreasing timing aversion. *Social Science and Medicine*, **45**, 1653–1659.
Cairns JA and van der Pol MM (1999) Do people value their own future health differently from others' future health? *Medical Decision Making*, **19**, 466–472.
Cairns JA and van der Pol MM (2000) The estimation of marginal time preference in a UK-wide sample (TEMPUS) project. *Health Technology Assessment*, **4**(1).
Cairns JA and van der Pol MM (2001) *Discrete choice with repeated follow-up: a web-based experiment*. HEB Working Paper 30, University of Bergen (http://129.177.180.16/heb/artikkel30.pdf).
Cameron TA (1988) A new paradigm for valuing non-market goods using referendum data: maximum likelihood estimation by censored logistic regression. *Journal of Environmental Economics and Management*, **15**, 355–379.

Cameron TA and Quiggin J (1994) Estimation using contingent valuation data from a dichotomous choice with follow-up. *Journal of Environmental Economics and Management*, **27**, 218–234.

Carson RT (1997) Contingent valuation: advances and empirical tests since the NOAA panel. *American Journal of Agricultural Economics*, **79**, 1501–1507.

Carson RT (2000) Contingent Valuation: a user's guide. *Environmental Science and Technology*, **34**, 1413–1418.

Chapman GB (1996) Temporal discounting and utility for health and money. *Journal of Experimental Psychology*, **22**, 771–791.

Chapman GB and Coups EJ (1999) Time preferences and preventive health behavior: acceptance of the influenza vaccine. *Medical Decision Making*, **19**, 307–314.

Chapman GB and Elstein AS (1995) Valuing the future: temporal discounting of health and money. *Medical Decision Making*, **15**, 373–386.

Chapman GB, Nelson R and Hier DB (1999) Familiarity and time preferences: decision making about treatments for migraine headaches and Crohn's disease. *Journal of Experimental Psychology: Applied*, **5**, 17–34.

Cooper JC (1993) Optimal bid design for dichotomous choice contingent valuation surveys. *Journal of Environmental Economics and Management*, **24**, 25–40.

Cropper ML, Aydede SK and Portney PR (1991) Discounting human lives. *American Journal of Agricultural Economics*, **73**, 1410–1415.

Cropper ML, Aydede SK and Portney PR (1994) Preferences for life saving programs: how the public discounts time and age. *Journal of Risk and Uncertainty*, **8**, 243–265.

Dolan P and Gudex C (1995) Time preference, duration and health state valuations. *Health Economics*, **4**, 289–299.

Enemark U, Lyttkens CH, Troeng T, Weibull H and Ranstam J (1998) Implicit discount rates of vascular surgeons in the management of abdominal aortic aneurysms. *Medical Decision Making*, **18**, 168–177.

Fredericks S, Loewenstein G and O'Donoghue T. (2002) Time discounting and time preference: a critical review. *Journal of Economical Literature*, **40**, 351–401.

Gafni A (1995) Time in health: can we measure individuals "pure time preferences"? *Medical Decision Making*, **15**, 31–37.

Gafni A and Torrance GW (1984) Risk attitude and time preference in health. *Management Science*, **30**, 440–451.

Ganiats TG, Carson RT, Hamm RM, Cantor SB, Sumner W, Spann SJ, Hagen MD and Miller C (2000) Population-based time preferences for future health outcomes. *Medical Decision Making*, **20**, 263–270.

Gyrd-Hansen D (2002) Comparing the results of applying different methods of eliciting time preferences for health. *European Journal of Health Economics*, **3**, 10–16.

Gyrd-Hansen D and Søgaard J (1998) Discounting life-years: whither time preference? *Health Economics*, **7**, 121–127.

Halvorsen B and Sælensminde K (1998) Differences in willingness-to-pay estimates from open-ended and discrete-choice contingent valuation methods: the effects of heteroscedasticity. *Land Economics*, **74**, 262–282.

Hausman JA (1979) Individual discount rates and the purchase of and utilisation of energy-using durables. *Bell Journal of Economics*, **10**, 33–54.

Höjgård S, Enemark U, Lyytkens CH, Lindgren A, Troëng T and Weibull H (2002) Discounting and clinical decision making: physicians, the general public, and the management of asymptomatic abdominal aortic aneurysms. *Health Economics*, **11**, 355–370.

Horowitz JH and Carson RT (1990) Discounting statistical lives. *Journal of Risk and Uncertainty*, **3**, 403–413.

Johannesson M and Johansson PO (1996) The discounting of lives saved in future generations – some empirical results. *Health Economics*, **5**, 329–332.

Johannesson M and Johansson PO (1997a) The value of life extension and the marginal rate of time preference: a pilot study. *Applied Economic Letters*, **4**, 53–55.

Johannesson M and Johansson PO (1997b) Quality of life and the WTP for an increased life expectancy at an advanced age. *Journal of Public Economics*, **65**, 219–228.

Lang K and Ruud PA (1986) Returns to schooling, implicit discount rates and black–white wage differentials. *Reviews of Economics and Statistics*, **69**, 41–47.

Lazaro A, Barberan R and Rubio E (2001) Private and social time preferences for health and money: an empirical estimation. *Health Economics*, **10**, 351–356.

Lazaro A, Barberan R and Rubio E (2002) The economic evaluation of health programmes: why discount health consequences more than monetary consequences? *Applied Economics*, **34**, 339–350.

Lipscomb J (1989) Time preference for health in cost-effectiveness analysis. *Medical Care*, **27**, S233–S253.

Loewenstein G and Prelec D (1993) Preferences for sequences of outcomes. *Psychological Review*, **100**, 91–108.

MacKeigan LD, Larson LN, Draugalis JR, Bootman JL and Burns LR (1993) Time preference for health gains versus health losses. *PharmacoEconomics*, **3**, 374–386.

Olsen JA (1993) Time preferences for health gains: an empirical investigation. *Health Economics*, **2**, 257–265.

Olsen JA (1994) Persons vs years: two ways of eliciting implicit weights. *Health Economics*, **3**, 39–46.

Olson M and Bailey MJ (1981) Positive time preference. In MJ Bailey (Ed.), *Studies in Positive and Normative Economics*. Elgar, Cheltenham, pp. 107–131.

Payne JW, Bettman JR and Johnson EJ (1993) *The Adaptive Decision Maker*. Cambridge University Press, Cambridge.

Poulos C and Whittington D (2000) Time preferences for life-saving programs: evidence from six less developed countries. *Environmental Science & Technology*, **34**, 1445–1455.

Redelmeier DA and Heller DN (1993) Time preference in medical decision making and cost-effectiveness analysis. *Medical Decision Making*, **13**, 212–217.

Stavem K, Kristiansen IS and Olsen JA (2002) Association of time preference for health with age and disease severity. *European Journal of Health Economics*, **3**, 120–124.

Tversky A, Slovic P and Sattath S (1988) Contingent weighting in judgment and choice. *Psychological Review*, **95**, 371–384.

van der Pol MM and Cairns JA (1999) Individual time preferences for own health: an application of a dichotomous choice question with follow-up. *Applied Economics Letters*, **6**, 649–654.

van der Pol MM and Cairns JA (2001) Estimating time preferences for health using discrete choice experiments. *Social Science and Medicine*, **52**, 1459–1470.

Viscusi WK and Moore MJ (1989) Rates of time preference and valuations of the duration of life. *Journal of Public Economics*, **38**, 297–317.

4

Economic Evaluation for Decision-making

ALASTAIR GRAY
Health Economics Research Centre, University of Oxford

LUKE VALE
Health Economics Research Unit & Health Services Research Unit,
University of Aberdeen

INTRODUCTION

Decisions about the optimal provision of health care are complex and one of the many pieces of information required by decision-makers is information concerning efficiency. Health economists have increasingly come to recognize that economic evaluations need to be analysed and reported in particular ways in order to meet the requirements of decision-makers, and that this in turn frequently requires the use of a range of modelling techniques.

In economic evaluation, modelling may take many different forms. It may refer to analytical techniques to synthesize costs and benefits of alternative interventions. In this case modelling could be used to inform future research or to make the evaluation results more 'useful' for health policy. Alternatively, it may refer to attempts to derive information on aspects of an economic evaluation. For example, it may relate to the synthesis of evidence on clinical effectiveness and quality of life; or extrapolation from intermediate endpoints to final outcomes.

Surveys of modelling in economic evaluation have generally focused on designing, constructing, parameterizing and evaluating the main types of model used to represent disease processes in economic evaluation, including decision tree analyses, Markov models and Monte Carlo simulation. A good example is Kuntz and Weinstein (2001). In this chapter the focus is on a range

Advances in Health Economics. Edited by Anthony Scott, Alan Maynard and Robert Elliott.
© 2003 John Wiley & Sons, Ltd

of modelling applications that can help to increase the usefulness of individual and multiple economic evaluations to decision-makers, to improve study design, and to inform the research agenda.

The first section of the chapter deals with measuring effectiveness in economic evaluation. It begins by drawing a distinction between intermediate endpoints and endpoints of more relevance to decision-makers who face multiple competing uses for the resources available. It then considers ways in which quality of life data can be translated into a form appropriate for economic evaluation. Finally, this section considers the synthesis of data from multiple sources to provide more comprehensive and precise estimates of clinical effects or quality of life.

The second section considers how economic evaluations can be made more relevant to decision-makers. It does this by focusing on one of the problems they face in this respect: the need to simulate the treatment comparisons that decision-makers are likely to be interested in, by synthesizing data from different sources.

Section three of the chapter considers the relevance of the total cost in the decision-making process, and the fourth section examines methods for making policy decisions using information from several economic evaluations of different interventions. In particular, the use of stochastic cost-effectiveness league tables, and the possible interactions between interventions. The fifth section of the chapter explores ways in which economists can contribute to decisions about the research agenda by reviewing expected value of perfect information (EVPI) analysis as a method of determining whether further research is required.

The chapter concludes by briefly highlighting implications for policy-makers of the techniques described and suggesting areas for further research.

MEASURING EFFECTIVENESS IN COST-EFFECTIVENESS ANALYSIS

How useful cost-effectiveness analysis (CEA) is in aiding resource allocation is related to the number of alternative ways resources could be employed. Consequently, a measure is required that can incorporate all relevant outcomes over the widest possible number of disease areas and interventions. At present, the main candidates for this are life years gained and quality adjusted life years (QALYs) gained, but many clinical studies use other measures of effectiveness, prompting a question about how they should be dealt with in cost-effectiveness analyses.

EXTRAPOLATION FROM INTERMEDIATE OR SURROGATE ENDPOINTS

Outcome measures can be classified hierarchically in terms of surrogate and clinical endpoints, mortality and morbidity, life expectancy and quality adjusted life expectancy. Typical surrogate endpoints are blood pressure, blood glucose or blood lipid levels; each is known to be an important risk factor for disease manifested in non-fatal or fatal endpoints such as myocardial infarction or stroke. The advantage of these measures is that differences can be measured in a relatively short time compared with the time required to identify differences in clinical endpoints. Therefore the cost of interventional studies is significantly reduced.

However, taking surrogate endpoints in CEA raises a number of problems. First, they restrict comparison to other interventions affecting the same surrogate endpoint. Second, as Johannesson *et al.* (1996) pointed out, comparing cost-effectiveness in terms of surrogate endpoints assumes that each unit of the surrogate measure has an equivalent value or effect on the health outcome of interest. This may not be the case – the relationship could be non-linear – while if the relationship is known it would be better to model the actual health outcome of interest instead (Johannesson *et al.* 1996). Thus, although some guidelines have at times advocated the use of surrogate endpoints in CEA on grounds of transparency and ease of clinical interpretation (Anonymous 1995), their use is generally not recommended.

Clinical endpoints (for example the incidence of coronary heart disease events, or cancer recurrences, or respiratory infections) may have an associated immediate and longer-term mortality rate, may reduce short-term and/or long-term quality of life, and may have an impact on the likelihood of experiencing further endpoints. As the relation between endpoints and final health outcomes (e.g. quality adjusted life expectancy) is likely to be highly variable, it seems clear that the cost per endpoint averted is of limited use and that modelling should be used to establish the link between surrogate endpoints and the time-dependent risk of experiencing a clinical endpoint, and thence the link between these endpoints and subsequent mortality and morbidity.

Survival as an outcome measure suffers from many of the same deficiencies as clinical endpoints: for example, a five-year survival rate counts as equivalent patients who survived one or four years, and likewise patients who survived six or 15 years. Wright and Weinstein (1998) argue that the use of gains in median survival time or gains in survival probability at a particular point in time (e.g. five-year survival), as shown in Figure 4.1, captures only one dimension of the shift in the survival curve and is potentially misleading compared to measuring the area between the two survival curves – that is, gain in life expectancy. Analysts should therefore make efforts to model and report gains in life

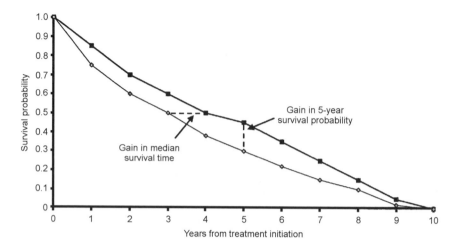

Figure 4.1 Hypothetical survival curves showing gain in median survival time, gain in five-year survival probability, and separation of survival curves corresponding to gain in life expectancy

expectancy from other intermediate or shorter-term endpoints (Wright & Weinstein 1998).

Following from this, if the intervention has a significant impact on quality of life, for example by reducing the number of non-fatal events that cause disability, or by prolonging survival in states of impaired quality of life, it is necessary to model quality adjusted life expectancy, by assigning a quality of life weight to each time period in each health state: e.g. (a) no heart disease, (b) non-fatal myocardial infarction, and (c) history of heart disease.

Finally, it is worth noting that many prospective CEAs performed alongside clinical trials will have access to information on clinical endpoints and/or surrogate endpoints and will also be following a study design that includes a commitment to estimate life years gained or quality adjusted life years gained as a final outcome measure. In these circumstances it is possible that significant differences exist in the surrogate endpoint but no significant difference is detected in the final outcome measure, especially where uncertainty has been fully addressed in the modelling process. It is also possible (if less likely) that individually non-significant differences in a number of surrogate endpoints may cumulatively cause a significant difference in final outcome. These and other circumstances will be encountered and remain to be resolved as experience in this area accumulates. However, for these and other reasons (in particular, the fact that most trials are not powered to test for equivalence) the decision to perform a CEA should not in general be conditioned on whether or not a trial demonstrates a difference in clinical effect.

QUALITY OF LIFE FOR ECONOMIC EVALUATION

Many clinical trials and observational studies now include health-related quality of life measures, including disease-specific instruments, generic health profiles, and preference or utility-based measures. The costs of including a full battery of instruments may be prohibitive to both investigators and participants, and may reduce response rates. If preference-based measures (or instruments like the EQ 5D that are underpinned by preference-based measures) are not included, then subsequent retrospective CEA may be limited. For these reasons, and in order to compare the validity, reliability, precision and responsiveness of different measures, there has been increasing interest in mapping responses from generic health profiles to health state preferences. One of the main generic health profile measures used in clinical trials is the SF-36, and to date five studies have reported algorithms that permit SF-36 responses to be converted to health state preference values (Fryback *et al.* 1997; Brazier *et al.* 1998, 2002; Shmueli 1998; Lundberg *et al.* 1999).

There are significant differences of approach between these studies. Fryback *et al.* (1997) reported an empirical equation allowing prediction of Quality of Well-Being (QWB) scores from the SF-36, using SF-36 and QWB responses collected by face-to-face interview from 1430 persons during the Beaver Dam Health Outcomes Study. They obtained a six-variable regression equation drawing on five of the eight SF-36 subscales to predict observed QWB variance. Shmueli adopted a similar approach, but used all eight SF-36 subscale scores and the visual analogue scale (VAS) responses from a sample of 1918 Israelis interviewed face-to-face as a measure of preference (*note*: the VAS is non-choice-based and is not unanimously considered to be preference-based).

Lundberg *et al.* (1999) asked a random population sample of 5404 Swedish adults by postal questionnaire to report their own current health using a visual analogue scale, a time trade-off (TTO) procedure and the SF-12 subset of the SF-36. The relationship between SF-12 responses and VAS and TTO responses was then estimated using full and reduced-form regression models.

Brazier *et al.* (1998) proceeded by converting the eight subscales of the SF-36 into a six-dimensional instrument (the SF-6D). They asked a convenience sample to place valuations using standard gamble (SG) and VAS on 59 of the possible 9000 health states generated by the SF-6D, and then used multiple regression to map SF-6D responses to the valuations. Finally, Brazier *et al.* (2002) reported the results of a similar exercise but with a larger general population sample of 611, a revised version of the SF-6D, and a valuation of 249 of 18,000 possible health states using standard gamble.

Of these five algorithms the ones by Fryback *et al.* (1997) and Shmueli (1998) could in principle be applied to published summary data on SF-36 subscale scores, but all the other algorithms require access to patient-level data.

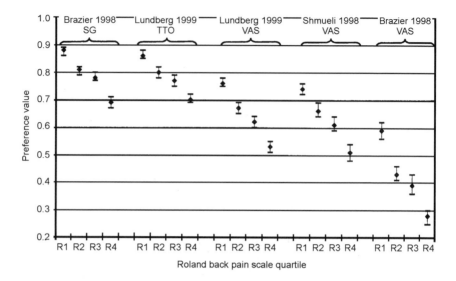

Figure 4.2 Relationship between mean (95% CI) preference values derived from various algorithms and quartiles of the Roland back pain scale
Source: Derived from Hollingworth *et al.* (2002), table 4

Hollingworth *et al.* (2002), reporting the results of a survey of 379 patients enrolled in a low back pain trial to whom the SF-36, VAS and TTO as well as a disease-specific back pain scale (modified Roland Scale) were administered, provide some comparative information on the performance of some of these algorithms. As Figure 4.2 shows, in all cases the predicted preference valuation decreased with increasing disease severity as indicated by the disease-specific instrument. In addition, the level of agreement between the two choice-based preference valuations for any level of disease severity was good, although there was less agreement between the non-choice-based valuations.

The modelling methods used to derive these algorithms have not yet been fully appraised, and it is not yet clear whether a correspondence between the health state valuations indicated by these algorithms and directly elicited valuations can be reproduced consistently in different studies. In addition, it is apparent that none of the choice-based algorithms is capable of generating a full range of quality of life valuations, with minimum values often in the region of 0.4 or higher, although this may be due to limitations of the SF-36 in defining severe health states as well as problems with the algorithms *per se*. However, these algorithm-based approaches do offer the prospect of modelling preference-based valuations of health states in circumstances where direct measures are not available, and therefore interest in their applications is likely to grow.

IMPROVING PRECISION OF CLINICAL EFFECT SIZES

One of the arguments advanced in the clinical literature to support the use of systematic reviews and meta-analysis of the available evidence is that decisions should be based upon evidence that is systematically assembled and analysed. While these arguments are most frequently made with respect to effectiveness, they can also be made with respect to cost-effectiveness. This is illustrated by Coyle and Lee (2002), who compared the cost-effectiveness of the bisphosphonate, alendronate, with no treatment as a method of preventing hip fractures. In their analysis they compared the results obtained when data from individual trials were compared to data from the meta-analysis. A cost-effectiveness acceptability curve (CEAC) was constructed for the different data sources. A CEAC is a graphical representation of the percentage of replications within a simulation exercise (in this case 5000 iterations of a Monte Carlo simulation), where the incremental cost per QALY is below a specific threshold. Using the results from two of the trials substantially underestimates the mean cost per QALY (Liberman *et al.* 1995; Black *et al.* 1996), while using the results of the third overestimates the mean cost per QALY. More importantly, the CEAC for the individual trials crosses that of the pooled estimates, indicating the greater uncertainty surrounding their results (Figure 4.3).

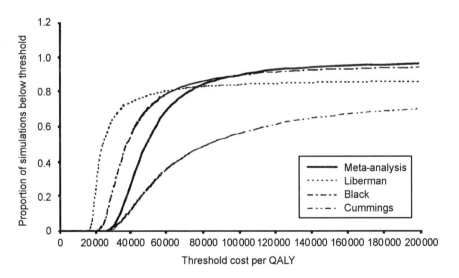

Figure 4.3 Cumulative distributions of cost per QALY for alendronate

MAKING THE ECONOMIC EVALUATION LOCALLY
RELEVANT: MODELLING TREATMENT COMPARISONS

The primary data available to decision-makers comes from comparisons between alternative treatments, new treatments vs. usual care, or treatment vs. placebo. Such data may not be immediately useful to decision-makers as they have to choose between mutually exclusive treatment options – for example, which ACE-inhibitor or beta blocker to prescribe for patients with hypertension – which few trials have directly compared. In these circumstances, health economists may have to extract information from a number of controlled trials each comparing one treatment option with a control or placebo, and use some form of modelling approach to estimate incremental cost-effectiveness. For example, Huse *et al.* (1998), recognizing the absence of large head-to-head outcome trials of cholesterol-lowering therapies, compared the cost-effectiveness of a range of statins by taking the results of a number of smaller trials that had made head-to-head comparisons between different statins using surrogate endpoints (effect of therapy on lipid levels), and then extrapolated to final outcomes using a heart disease risk equation within a Markov model. This approach retained the benefits of using randomization to avoid bias, but had the disadvantages of relying on short-term data using intermediate outcomes.

An alternative approach was adopted by van Hoot and Simoons (2001), who combined within a model the cardiovascular risk reduction results from five separate long-term outcome trials that had each compared a statin against a control arm, in order to compare cost-effectiveness for a range of population groups with different levels of initial risk. A third approach was taken by O'Brien *et al.* (1994), who attempted a more direct comparison of two alternative therapies for the prophylaxis of deep vein thrombosis by extracting data from the treatment arms of 10 randomized trials which had each compared one or other therapy against placebo, pooling the event and cost variables, and then estimating incremental cost-effectiveness. However, this approach has been criticized by Bucher *et al.* (1997), who argue that variations in the populations from which these trials were drawn leave the results subject to bias and mean that the benefits of randomization have been lost. They propose instead a method based on direct comparison of the magnitude of treatment effects of interventions compared to control groups in the available trials, but acknowledge that this will not protect against all possible biases.

The techniques set out above all make use of summary data from published studies. Another potential way of modelling direct comparisons of cost-effectiveness between treatment options in the absence of trial comparisons would be to obtain and pool patient-level data from different trials, thereby permitting direct comparison of different interventions while controlling for baseline differences in risk factors relating to different trial populations, entry criteria and randomization processes. This approach is currently being pursued for clinical outcomes using data from all ongoing or planned large-scale randomized trials of cholesterol treatment in the Cholesterol Treatment Trialists' (CTT) Collaboration, and similar approaches embracing outcome and resource use variables are under development in a number of treatment areas.

THE RELEVANCE OF TOTAL COST

It is now generally accepted that research funding agencies such as the National Health Service Health Technology Assessment programme and the Medical Research Council will frequently require the inclusion of economic evaluations in the randomized controlled trials they fund. Guidelines for the design, conduct and presentation of such studies are well established (Drummond & Jefferson 1996; NICE 2000b). However, these guidelines focus primarily on the accurate estimation of a cost-effectiveness ratio using specified methods to handle costs, outcomes and uncertainty. Decision-makers may or may not make use of cost-effectiveness ratios when deciding on the introduction of a new technology, but insofar as they do they will frequently also be concerned with the total cost and service implications of introducing the technology. For example, the Department of Health and Treasury are not indifferent to the total cost impact of some treatment recommendation incorporated in a National Service Framework, even if it has a favourable cost-effectiveness ratio.

ASSESSING BUDGETARY IMPACT

Figure 4.4 shows the total expenditure of a hypothetical primary care trust on a set of independent and indivisible interventions, arranged in order of ascending cost-effectiveness with the width of each bar indicating the total cost of each intervention. Cumulative expenditure is just under £1m. It is evident that, within this budget constraint, the opportunity cost of displacing existing interventions increases as the total cost of the new intervention rises, because the least cost-effective existing services will, or at least should, be displaced first to make way for more cost-effective alternatives. Consequently, it is necessary to consider a new intervention's cost-effectiveness and total cost jointly. Some agencies do require analysts to give an indication of the likely 'budget impact' of a technology (NICE 2000b), but the methodologies to be used are not specified and no distinction is drawn between financial costs and economic (opportunity) costs, which in certain circumstances could differ markedly. In turn, estimation of the total cost of an intervention focuses attention on the

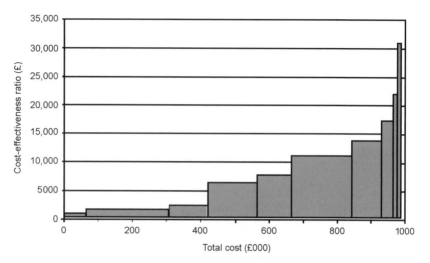

Figure 4.4 Allocation of a fixed budget to interventions by total cost and cost-effectiveness ratio

true indivisibility of that intervention, and the degree of variation in cost-effectiveness within it.

Estimating the total costs and benefits associated with an intervention is also relevant to the increasing interest in assessing the value of obtaining information from additional research. In that framework, information has value insofar as it reduces the costs of uncertainty surrounding a decision, and these costs depend in turn on the size of the patient population and its capacity to benefit. This issue is considered in more detail below.

ECONOMIC EVALUATION AND MULTIPLE INTERVENTIONS

While the literature on handling uncertainty in the estimation of cost-effectiveness has grown rapidly in recent years, it has focused primarily on uncertainty concerning the cost-effectiveness of individual interventions. Relatively little attention has been paid to how decision-makers should make use of cost-effectiveness information on a number of interventions, all of which may potentially be of interest. For example, the confidence intervals surrounding the cost-effectiveness ratios of different interventions may overlap, with no interventions unambiguously superior to alternatives. Or, interventions may not be truly independent; or there may be scope for joint production of different interventions, for example by providing clinics intended to deal with multiple risk factors for heart disease.

QALY LEAGUE TABLES AND UNCERTAINTY

The standard assumption concerning cost-effectiveness league tables is that interventions are ranked in order of the point-estimate of cost-effectiveness, and decision-makers then work down the list until the budget constraint is reached [we acknowledge but are not directly concerned here with other problems of cost-effectiveness league tables, such as methodological differences between studies (Gerard & Mooney 1993)].

This approach rank orders interventions by expected value and ignores the variance surrounding the point-estimates of cost-effectiveness. By doing so, it implicitly assumes that decision-makers are indifferent to risk, but previous analyses using the framework of portfolio theory have shown that health care managers may well be risk-averse and will wish to include risk characteristics when selecting a portfolio of investments in different interventions (O'Brien & Sculpher 2000). Thus, the general failure to integrate uncertainty into the decision-making process is a potentially serious problem.

One proposed method for incorporating uncertainty into the cost-effectiveness results presented to decision-makers is to construct *stochastic league tables*. To do so requires the assembly of information on the total costs and total effects of each intervention and the variance around costs and effects. Random draws are then taken from the estimated distribution of costs and effects for each intervention, the appropriate cost-effectiveness ratio is calculated, the interventions are ordered according to cost-effectiveness, and those falling within the budget constraint are recorded. The process is then repeated a large number of times to give a stable estimate of the probability that each intervention will fall within the budget constraint. Table 4.1 gives an illustration of this, with 11 interventions in three mutually exclusive sets A, B and C. Each cost and effect pair is subject to variance (not shown), and so cost-effectiveness will vary around the point-estimates shown, while in some circumstances the comparator will also change within a mutually exclusive set. At a budget constraint of 50, there is a 43% probability that intervention C1 will fall within the budget constraint, but as the budget constraint is relaxed the preferred intervention will switch to C2 and then C3. When the budget constraint rises to 200, a second intervention B2 can be admitted, and so on.

The stochastic league table approach has not yet been demonstrated in a real decision-making environment, and a number of limitations may arise. First, it is not clear how the approach would work in circumstances where scores or even hundreds of potential interventions could be selected. Second, it is not clear to what extent the approach captures the costs of changing from one intervention to another as the budget expands, but it is at least questionable that decision-makers, clinicians or patients would be prepared to accept frequent policy changes as suggested in the expansion paths of Table 4.1. Third, by presenting information probabilistically, the approach makes it

ADVANCES IN HEALTH ECONOMICS

Table 4.1 Costs, effects and cost-effectiveness of three independent sets of mutually exclusive interventions (A, B and C), and probability of inclusion of interventions in optimal mix at different budget constraints

Intervention	Total cost	Total effect	Incremental cost-effectiveness[a]	Budget constraint							
				50	100	150	200	300	400	600	800
A1	120	1	—	0	0	0	0	1	2	0	0
A2	140	5.5	25.4	0	0	1	1	5	25	28	29
A3	170	3	—	0	0	0	0	0	1	4	4
A4	190	7	33.3	0	0	0	0	0	11	67	67
B1	100	12	—	0	3	14	11	2	0	0	0
B2	120	17	7.1	0	1	18	35	26	21	15	15
B3	150	20	10.0	0	0	4	36	72	78	85	85
C1	50	22	2.3	43	40	30	36	8	3	0	0
C2	70	24.5	8.0	14	47	25	37	17	10	0	0
C3	120	29	11.1	0	13	38	16	45	33	24	23
C4	170	31	25.0	0	0	8	11	31	54	76	76

[a] Incremental cost-effectiveness ratios calculated after dominated interventions excluded.

easier to assess the trade-offs between efficiency objectives and other policy objectives: for example, at a budget constraint of 200, the probability of B3 being in the optimum mix of interventions is 36%, while the probability of B2 being included is 35%. On efficiency grounds B3 would be preferred, but the efficiency loss arising from selecting B2 would be small. However, this assessment of trade-off can only be performed within mutually exclusive sets of interventions, where much of the policy interest may concern trade-off between independent interventions. And fourth, the information requirements of the approach are relatively heavy: information on variance around costs and effects (and covariance) are frequently not presented in a form suitable for this type of analysis, and information on the total costs and effects of interventions, as noted earlier in this chapter, is less easy to produce than is commonly thought.

The relationship between stochastic league tables and other approaches to similar or related problems also remains to be explored, in particular, the portfolio approach to resource allocation, the use of multiple cost-effectiveness acceptability curves, the net benefit approach and stochastic frontier analysis.

INTERACTION BETWEEN INTERVENTIONS

The stochastic league table approach, and the budget impact analyses discussed in the previous section, are premised on the indivisibility of the interventions considered, and also assume that non-mutually exclusive interventions are genuinely independent in their costs and effects. This may not be the case. For example, it is possible to assess separately the cost-effectiveness of improved glycaemic control and improved blood pressure control amongst hypertensive type 2 diabetic patients. However, it is quite possible that at least some of the nurse and doctor consultations required to provide these interventions could be combined and provided at less than the additive cost, breaking the independence assumption.

Similarly, the simultaneous adoption of a set of independent interventions may produce interactions in health effects: full implementation of all cost-effective interventions for coronary heart disease, for example, may have an appreciable effect on the absolute risk of coronary heart disease, suggesting that the effect of each intervention should be considered as multiplicative (independent) rather than additive.

INFORMING THE RESEARCH AGENDA

The data available to decision-makers are often limited and as a result decisions are made not only about the adoption of the intervention(s) under investigation but also about whether to conduct further research and so reduce the uncertainty in the decision-making process. The funds available for such research are limited and decisions have to be made about what research should be undertaken.

In earlier sections of this chapter it was argued that decision-makers would not be indifferent to the uncertainty surrounding estimates of cost-effectiveness of alternative interventions; similarly it cannot be expected that decision-makers will be indifferent to the products of research. As briefly mentioned earlier, one way to characterize the nature of this uncertainty is the use of probabilistic analysis which facilitates the adoption of a value of information approach (Claxton & Posnett 1996), and which can then be used to identify future research options.

ASSESSING THE VALUE OF FURTHER RESEARCH

Fenwick *et al.* (2000) considered a Bayesian value of information approach to consider the potential costs of uncertainty in decisions about the management of urinary tract infections in order to estimate the value of additional information and the most efficient way of obtaining it. In their analysis the expected value of perfect information (EVPI) was taken as being equal to the expected costs of uncertainty surrounding a decision on service delivery made using currently available information. They were able to show EVPI for different values of a unit of health gain for the different strategies they considered and for the different parameters included in the model. For example they showed that the value of EVPI for prevalence of urinary tract symptoms was quite low, while further information about side-effects of treatment and utilities had the greatest value.

DETERMINING THE NATURE OF FUTURE RESEARCH

Value of information analyses such as that by Fenwick *et al.* allow the identification of the most crucial parameters for future work. In particular they allow the consideration of the cost uncertainty in the analysis as a whole rather than uncertainty surrounding individual parameters, which is all traditional deterministic models relying on one-way sensitivity analysis can investigate. Knowledge of the key determinants of costs, effects and cost-effectiveness can be used to help determine the type of future study.

Where the key determinant of cost-effectiveness is relative effectiveness, then the appropriate study design to obtain more precise and less biased estimates of the key determinants of costs, effects and cost-effectiveness might be a randomized control trial. In some circumstances such information might more appropriately be obtained from an observational study. In a recent evaluation of metal-on-metal hip arthroplasty one of the most important parameters was the rate of failure of this operation in the long term, as this was a principal determinant of QALYs and data were sparse (Vale *et al.* 2002). Given the comparative rarity of this outcome it was felt that the most appropriate study design would be a population-based registry (NICE 2000a). Fenwick *et al.* noted in their study that for the parameters where the value of information was the greatest (utilities and side-effects) an RCT would not be appropriate and less expensive non-experimental designs would be more appropriate.

CONCLUSIONS

Decision-makers face a difficult task in allocating the scarce resources available to them. Economic evaluation has the potential to assist decision-makers by providing a framework to combine disparate pieces of information that individually may have limited use. It can also assist decision-makers by exploring and quantifying the nature and extent of the uncertainty they face.

In particular the need to make comparisons between interventions has led economists to adopt and adapt techniques to extrapolate data from more limited outcome measures (surrogate endpoints or non-preference-based measures of quality of life). Such approaches may allow comparisons to be made on the basis of a common measure of outcome, e.g. QALYs.

Such approaches will not, by themselves, be sufficient for policy-makers. Decisions often have to be made using information that is subject to some degree of imprecision or does not directly relate to the decision to be made. The use of techniques to 'pool' information from multiple sources can increase the precision of estimates of cost-effectiveness as well as allow the modelling of indirect comparisons. There may still be considerable uncertainty around estimates of costs, effects and cost-effectiveness which decision-makers will not be indifferent to. The use of stochastic techniques should, arguably, assist decision-makers as they can be used to characterize this uncertainty and so facilitate decisions about which services to provide and what further research to undertake.

Although the techniques described in this chapter could be of great value to decision-makers, the theory and application of all require further research. One area of further research relates to the modelling of final outcomes (for example, cost per QALYs) from surrogate endpoints. Although it has been argued in this chapter that this would be desirable, more experience is needed in understanding the relationships between surrogate outcomes and final outcomes. Similarly, more research is required on the use of algorithms to convert health profiles into health state preferences, in particular to confirm consistency of valuations between different studies and to overcome limitations in valuing severe health states.

Handling the uncertainty surrounding estimates of cost, effects and cost-effectiveness has received much attention in the last few years and considerable progress has been made in the use of stochastic techniques. However, further research is now required to determine which if any of the innovations such as stochastic league tables, the portfolio approach to resource allocation, multiple cost-effectiveness acceptability curves, the net benefit approach and stochastic frontier analysis will be of most use to decision-makers having to choose packages of interventions from fixed budgets.

Finally, although several areas of further research have been highlighted above, we would stress that the techniques discussed in this chapter already have the potential (although further research would increase their usefulness) to assist policy-makers in the very real and difficult problems of resource allocation, and using them need not be conditional on this research being performed.

ACKNOWLEDGEMENTS

The authors are grateful to Andy Briggs and David Parkin and participants at the HERU workshop for comments on an earlier draft. HERU is funded by the Chief Scientist Office of the Scottish Executive Health Department. The views are those of the authors.

REFERENCES

Anonymous (1995) *Guidelines for the pharmaceutical industry on preparation of submission to the Pharmaceutical Benefits Advisory Committee, including economic analyses.* Commonwealth of Australia, Department of Human Services and Health. Australia Government Publishing Service, Canberra.

Black DM, Cummings SR, Karpf DB, Cauley JA, Thompson DE, Nevitt MC *et al.* (1996) Randomised trial of effect of alendronate on risk of fracture in women with existing vertebral fractures. Fracture Intervention Trial Research Group. *Lancet*, **348**, 1535–1541.

Brazier J, Usherwood T, Harper R and Thomas K (1998) Deriving a preference-based single index from the UK SF-36 Health Survey. *Journal of Clinical Epidemiology*, **51**, 1115–1128.

Brazier J, Roberts J and Deverill M (2002) The estimation of a preference-based measure of health from the SF-36. *Journal of Health Economics*, **21**, 271–292.

Bucher H, Guyatt G, Griffith L and Walter S (1997) The results of direct and indirect treatment comparisons in meta-analysis of randomised controlled trials. *Journal of Clinical Epidemiology*, **50**(6), 683–691.

Claxton K and Posnett J (1996) An economic approach to clinical trial design and research priority-setting. *Health Economics*, **5**, 513–524.

Coyle D and Lee K (2002) Evidence based economic evaluation: how the use of different data sources can impact results. In C Donaldson, M Mugford and L Vale (Eds), *From Effectiveness to Efficiency – Health Economics and Systematic Review*. BMJ Books, London.

Drummond MF and Jefferson T on behalf of the BMJ Economic Evaluation Working Party (1996) Guidelines for authors and peer reviewers of economic submissions to the BMJ. *British Medical Journal*, **313**, 275–283.

Fenwick E, Claxton K, Sculpher M and Briggs A (2000) *Improving the efficiency and relevance of health technology assessment: the role of iterative decision analytic modelling*. The University of York, Centre for Health Economics, Discussion Paper 179.

Fryback DG, Lawrence WF, Martin PA, Klein R and Klein BEK (1997) Predicting quality of well-being scores from the SF-36: Results from the Beaver Dam Health Outcomes Study. *Medical Decision Making*, **17**, 1–9.

Gerard K and Mooney G (1993) QALY league tables: handle with care. *Health Economics*, **2**, 59–64.

Hollingworth W, Deyo R, Sullivan S, Emerson S, Gray D and Jarvik J (2002) The practicality and validity of directly elicited and SF-36 derived health state preferences in patients with low back pain. *Health Economics*, **11**, 71–85.

Huse DM, Russell MW, Miller JD, Kraemer DF, D'Agostino RB, Ellison RC and Hartz SC (1998) Cost-effectiveness of statins. *American Journal of Cardiology*, **82**, 1357–1363.

Johannesson M, Jonsson B and Karlsson G (1996) Outcome measurement in economic evaluation. *Health Economics*, **5**, 279–296.

Kuntz K and Weinstein M (2001) Modelling in economic evaluation. In M Drummond and A McGuire (Eds), *Economic Evaluation in Health Care: Merging Theory with Practice*. Oxford University Press, Oxford, pp. 141–170.

Liberman UA, Weiss SR, Broll J, Minne HW, Quan H, Bell NH, Rodriguez-Portales J, Downs RW Jr, Dequeker J and Favus M (1995) Effect of oral alendronate on bone mineral density and the incidence of fractures in postmenopausal osteoporosis. The Alendronate Phase III Osteoporosis Treatment Study Group. *New England Journal of Medicine*, **333**, 1437–1443.

Lundberg L, Johannesson M, Isacson DG and Borgquist L (1999) The relationship between health-state utilities and the SF-12 in a general population. *Medical Decision Making*, **19**, 128–140.

NICE (National Institute for Clinical Excellence) (2000a) *Appraisal Consultation Document; Metal on metal hip resurfacing arthroplasty.* www.nice.org.uk/pdf/hipsmo macdnocomments.pdf

NICE (National Institute for Clinical Excellence) (2000b) *Guidance for manufacturers and sponsors. Technology Appraisal Process No. 5.* www.nice.org.uk/pdf/technical guidanceformanufacturersandsponsors.pdf

O'Brien BJ and Sculpher MJ (2000) Building uncertainty into cost-effectiveness rankings: portfolio risk–return tradeoffs and implications for decision rules. *Medical Care*, **38**(5), 460–468.

O'Brien B, Anderson DT and Goeree R (1994) Cost-effectiveness of enoxaparin versus warfarin prophylaxis against deep-vein thrombosis after total hip replacement. *Canadian Medical Association Journal*, **150**, 1083–1090.

Schulman KA, Buxton M, Glick H, Sculpher M, Guzman G, Kong J, Backhouse M, Mauskopf J, Bell L and Eisenberg JM (1996) Results of the economic evaluation of the first study. A multinational prospective economic evaluation. FIRST Investigators. Flolan International Randomized Survival Trial. *International Journal of Technological Assessments in Health Care*, **12**, 698–713.

Shmueli A (1998) The SF-36 profile and health-related quality of life: an interpretative analysis. *Quality of Life Research*, **7**, 187–195.

Vale L, Wyness L, McCormack K, McKenzie L, Brazzelli M and Stearns S (2002) Systematic review of the effectiveness and cost-effectiveness of metal on metal hip resurfacing arthroplasty for treatment of hip disease. *Health Technology Assessment*, **6**(15), 1–109.

van Hoot B and Simoons M (2001) Cost-effectiveness of HMG coenzyme reductase inhibitors; whom to treat? *European Heart Journal*, **22**(9), 751–761.

Wright JC and Weinstein MC (1998) Gains in life expectancy from medical interventions – standardizing data on outcomes. *New England Journal of Medicine*, **339**, 380–386.

5

Incentives in Health Care

ANTHONY SCOTT
Health Economics Research Unit, University of Aberdeen

SHELLEY FARRAR
Health Economics Research Unit, University of Aberdeen

INTRODUCTION

Market failures in health care mean that the incentives for behaviour change that exist in a competitive market cannot be relied upon to deliver improvements in efficiency in the health care market (Rice 2001). Exchange relationships within health care organizations, and between health care providers, patients and third-party payers, are characterized by asymmetry of information, a lack of consumer sovereignty and the subsequent development of agency relationships. These agency relationships have been at the centre of much debate and research within health economics and are key in discussions about the role of incentives in the health care sector.

The traditional focus of agency problems in health care has been supplier-induced demand (SID) and the effects of competition and financial incentives for doctors (Labelle *et al.* 1994; McGuire 2000). There are many reviews of the effects of different payment systems and incentives on doctors' behaviour (Hellinger 1996; McGuire 2000; Gosden *et al.* 2001). Other studies have focused directly on the doctor–patient relationship itself and the role of information transmission and decision-making within it, as a potential solution to agency problems at this level (Vick & Scott 1998; Scott & Vick 1999).

Agency problems have also been examined at different levels, including influencing the performance of hospitals and other health care organizations (Whynes 1993; Propper 1995; Chalkley & Malcolmson 1998; Hausman & LeGrand 1999; Goddard *et al.* 2000; Sloan 2000). Some of this literature is reviewed in Chapter 7. Considerations of agency problems have also led to

Advances in Health Economics. Edited by Anthony Scott, Alan Maynard and Robert Elliott.
© 2003 John Wiley & Sons, Ltd

research on the objectives of incentives schemes in terms of what patients value from health care, suggesting that it is this that needs to be specified first, before incentives can be designed to deliver it (Mooney & Ryan 1993).

The health economics literature has grown against the background of several developments in the economic theory of incentives. The aim of this chapter is to review these developments and examine how they apply to incentives for physicians and health care organizations in the UK. It is suggested that the focus of research in health economics on explicit incentive schemes based in agency theory is perhaps misplaced. It does so because there are many reasons why such incentives may not work as intended, and other types of implicit contracts are likely to play a greater role in influencing behaviour and performance.

In particular, a number of recent reviews of the literature on incentives in firms, within the fields of personnel and labour economics, are summarized. Work combining economic frameworks and models with theories in psychology and sociology that have been applied to the area of incentives is also reviewed. These theories have addressed the role of pecuniary and non-pecuniary sources of motivation. The relevance of these issues for the UK health care system is discussed, and further research is identified.

THE ECONOMICS OF INCENTIVES

In keeping with the mainstream economics literature on agency, the health economics literature has tended to focus on applications of basic agency problems and their solutions in the form of incentive contracts. However, in health care where physicians have a strong ethical interest in 'doing good' for their patients, it has been suggested that there is less need for strong external incentives (Mooney & Ryan 1993). Moreover, the UK health care system has few explicit incentive schemes for physicians, where they are either paid using mixed payment schemes that ameliorate the effects of any single payment scheme, or are paid by salary. For example, GPs are paid a mix of capitation payment, fee-for-service, flat rate payments and target payments, and hospital doctors are paid by salary. Hospital reimbursement in the UK (discussed more fully in Chapter 7) has also been characterized by the lack of strong external incentives.

The focus of research on explicit incentive contracts as a mechanism for changing behaviour and improving performance is perhaps misplaced in health economics, as there is a more general recognition that such schemes form only a small proportion of actual payment systems in practice. This is a message being put forward in several recent and major reviews of the economics literature on the provision of incentives in organizations (Gibbons 1997; Gibbons & Waldman 1999; Lazear 1999, 2000; Malcolmson 1999; Prendergast

1999). The literature has also been reviewed in the context of the public sector (Burgess & Metcalfe 1999a; Dixit 2001). Much of this work has been gathered under the banner of 'Personnel Economics', reflecting the application of economics to human resource issues that opens the 'black box' of the neoclassical firm (Lazear 2000). Although these reviews have unfortunately ignored the contribution of the health economics literature on incentives and agency (e.g. Mooney & Ryan 1993), it remains the case that these reviews contain ideas that have yet to be applied in health care settings.

These reviews cite a large body of empirical evidence that lends support to the assumptions and predictions of the basic principal–agent model: that financial incentives do matter, confirming the existence of monetary factors in individual utility functions; that pay varies with performance, confirming that firms believe individuals will respond to financial incentives and do employ these incentives within contracts. The authors of these reviews accept that the classic agency model is limited in a number of ways and that it cannot explain the deficiencies of the model when applied to the real world – in particular the evidence that performance-related pay can be counterproductive and inefficient, and that the use of explicit performance contracts is rare in practice. These deficiencies have led to many extensions of the basic agency model, and new avenues of theoretical and empirical research on incentives. The following sections summarize the main issues arising from the recent literature and how they apply to health care.

MULTITASKING

A main theme is that compensation schemes can have unintended consequences that are beneficial to agents but not to principals. The classic paper by Holmstrom and Milgrom (1991), and other models (Baker 1992), emphasize 'multitasking'. They distinguish between the agent's total contribution to a firm (y), and the agent's measured performance (p) (Gibbons & Waldman 1999). If a principal contracts on p rather than y, then the effect of such a contract depends on the correlation between the marginal effects of effort on p and y. When p omits important dimensions of y, the principals will 'get what they pay for', i.e. p and not y. When the agent has a complex job description that requires them to undertake many related tasks at once, i.e. 'multitasking', then y has many dimensions. The problem may be compounded if p is measured with error, and agents 'game' the compensation system for their own gain, i.e. where other outcomes exist that are valuable to the agent but not to the principal. Paying for performance does not necessarily lead to improvements in efficiency and can distort an agent's behaviour since they emphasize only those aspects of tasks that are rewarded. Complex jobs and organizations will not typically be rewarded through explicit contracts. This is one reason why performance pay is not commonly observed, even if there are a number of objective and specific performance measures available. A good example of this is the neglect of quality to reduce costs or increase profits (Dixit 2001), which is discussed in the context of hospital behaviour in Chapter 7.

There are many examples of such behaviour in health care, where jobs and tasks are complex and where a particular type of payment system encourages specific types of behaviours to the detriment of others. Examination of the effects of different systems of paying doctors has provided strong evidence that incentives operate as predicted, and that doctors may 'game' the system for their own gain.

For example, the evidence on the role of fee-for-service payment and capitation payment consistently highlights issues of over-treatment and 'cream-skimming' (McGuire 2000; Gosden et al. 2001). Empirical evidence of payment systems has not examined the opportunity costs of those behaviours that were encouraged as a result of the introduction of the financial incentive. For example, the introduction of payments for minor surgery to British GPs in 1991 encouraged more of this activity in primary care, but did not reduce the use of minor surgery in hospitals, suggesting that GPs' activity was additional to that conducted in hospitals (O'Cathain et al. 1992). The failure to examine the effect on other displaced activities means that the effect of fees and payments on efficiency is not known. Similarly, the 1990 GP contract also introduced target payments for cervical cytology and immunizations. Most GPs in the UK now hit these targets and so respond as expected, although again the opportunity costs of this activity are not known (Hughes & Yule 1992; Guiffrida et al. 2001).

The inherent difficulty in defining hospital output adds to the complexity of agency within the hospital sector. Looking only at health care per se, there are many different types of health care patients and treatments. Broadening to its full remit, the hospital is responsible for hotel services, teaching, research, laboratory services, etc. Hence the complex multi-output nature of hospital activity and the applicability of the multitask agency problem is clear. Preyra and Pink (2001) use the multitask principal–agent model to predict the differences in performance-related earnings of CEOs of profit and non-profit hospitals in the USA. Their results show that non-profit hospitals reward their CEOs less generously than for profit, but the CEOs in the for profit hospitals can expect greater variation in their pay, indicating a greater spread of rewards and thus stronger incentives. Preyra and Pink use this evidence to argue that high-powered incentives are more commonly used in for profit hospitals where the performance of the hospital and thus the CEO can be closely linked to a simple financial outcome measure in the form of surpluses or profit. The non-profit hospitals do not adopt such high-powered incentives, as they do not want the CEO to 'substitute effort away from less observable tasks'.

The abolition of the UK NHS internal market acknowledged a pre-existing gradual move away from the annual re-negotiation of contracts, towards the use of long-term service agreements. Nevertheless, there are still strong multitasking concerns as hospitals and other NHS organizations are now subject to specific performance targets following the development of national performance frameworks. The performance indicators are based on six (seven in Scotland) broad areas of outcome and activity (for example, health improvement, fair access, public involvement) and within these broad headings a plethora of specific performance indicators exist. Explicit weights are not attached to these performance criteria, theoretically giving them all equal importance. However, Goddard *et al.* (2000) in a qualitative study of 'unintended and dysfunctional behavioural consequences... of performance measures' report that the attention given to waiting times distracted attention away from other less easily measurable but important activities and outcomes.

SUBJECTIVE PERFORMANCE EVALUATION

A more common form of assessing performance in jobs is the use of subjective performance evaluation. This may be used extensively alongside salary payment, where promotions or the award of bonuses are dependent on a subjective assessment of the overall contribution to a firm (y) along numerous dimensions. It may therefore avoid the problems of multitasking. There is little empirical economics literature on this issue, although it has been the subject of theoretical models (Prendergast 1999).

The problem of these implicit contracts is that they cannot be easily verified by a third party. The principal may also have an incentive to under-report performance to save on wages and keep costs down, particularly if the principal is a residual claimant of firm profits. This may be more likely in firms subject to more competition. However, these problems may be overcome in a dynamic context as the principal would still want to encourage effort in future periods. Both explicit contracts (based on p) and implicit contracts (based on y) may also be used. The weight placed on the subjective measure increases in the noisiness (and relevance) of the objective performance measure (Baker *et al.* 1994a), although the empirical evidence of this is mixed (Burgess & Metcalfe 1999b; Prendergast 1999).

Inefficiency may also arise where principals distort individual ratings by not differentiating good performance from bad. This leads to 'centrality bias', where principals provide ratings that differ little around some norm, and 'leniency bias', where principals overstate the performance of poor performers to avoid the disutility of delivering 'bad news'. There may therefore be a trade-off between the provision of incentives for effort and the inefficiency of these biases. These problems may also be more severe where performance appraisals are linked to pay setting. Many firms explicitly separate performance appraisal from pay setting, although some subjective assessment of performance is still required for promotion.

Another form of bias is where agents undertake actions to increase the likelihood of a better rating from principals, where such actions have less value to the firm than other activities. In addition, 'currying favour' with principals may lead them to inflate performance ratings and exhibit favouritism. It then becomes difficult to determine 'true' performance. Prendergast (1999) comments on the paucity of economics literature examining subjectively assessed performance.

In health care, particularly in salaried jobs, subjective performance evaluation is commonplace and used in many contexts. In the UK NHS, this has been a feature of the majority of non-medical jobs. However, for both hospital doctors and GPs in the UK, annual performance appraisal did not exist prior to 2002. Nevertheless, other forms of subjective performance evaluation have existed for hospital consultants in determining whether they receive distinction awards. These are a form of bonus awarded to consultants for special contributions to medicine, exceptional ability or outstanding professional work – an emphasis is placed on prestige and reputation, which may not always be related to doing their job well from their employer's or the patients' perspectives. The highest award (A+) can almost double a consultant's salary.

Distinction awards have been heavily criticized in the past as they used to be awarded to consultants for life, and the process by which they were awarded was secret, dominated by other doctors and had no explicit or public criteria. There was little relationship between awards and crude measures of productivity (Bloor & Maynard 1992). In 1990, the system was reformed so that awards were reviewed after five years, there was more employer involvement on award committees, and age limits for new awards were imposed. Further changes were made in 1999. The potential inefficiencies outlined in the agency literature are clearly applicable here, including centrality and leniency bias. 'Currying favour' and undertaking actions that are beneficial to the consultant and not necessarily to patients or the hospital is also likely to be a problem, raising issues of favouritism and conflict of objectives. Additionally, since the subjective evaluation is directly linked to pay, these problems may be severe.

Subjective performance assessment has also been used at an organizational level. For example, in Scotland, each health authority's annual performance was monitored through its 'Accountability Review'. These took the form of ongoing bilateral discussions between the central government and health authorities on planned targets and actual performance as defined in the 'Corporate Contract' between the two parties. The health authorities were encouraged to use quantifiable outcome-based objectives in these contracts as the basis for a subjective assessment of overall performance. However, ultimately the health authority determined the objectives, and the ongoing discussions enabled them to draw on local circumstances to 'explain' shortfalls on targets. This is an example of the use of both explicit performance measures and implicit subjective performance.

INCENTIVES IN TEAMS

Teams are an integral part of the provision of health care services. The many different skills required in the treatment of specific episodes of health care mean that tasks undertaken by different health professionals have to be carefully integrated to produce high-quality health care. Incentives to enhance co-operation in team production are therefore important. However, economic theory on this issue focuses on external incentives and team rewards, whereas in health care there may be less need for strong incentives if health professionals' ethical interests motivate them to produce effort in a team environment.

The main issue with team production in economics, where output reflects the actions of many individuals and the team as a whole is rewarded, is free riding where workers may 'shirk' and produce less effort relative to others as the share of their reward is based on group effort, not individual effort.[1] There is much empirical evidence to support the existence of free riding in the general economic literature. One potential solution is the use of peer pressure and mutual monitoring, where its impact on efficiency depends on its costs and whether there are any rewards or punishments associated with monitoring. Studies that examine the effect of profit-sharing schemes show that productivity is higher under such schemes even when there are large numbers of workers, suggesting that the free-rider problem is not important. However, these studies may have flawed study designs and may not represent a strict test of the theory (Prendergast 1999; Lazear 2000).

Some studies have also shown that the use of team-based compensation improves the performance of the least productive team members, and reduces the performance of the most productive (Weiss 1987; Hansen 1997). Medium-ability workers are more likely to stay in the job, the best-ability workers leave because they prefer individual compensation schemes, while the least able leave because of peer pressure. The spread of ability of workers in a team is therefore important. It has also been found that a more compressed wage structure may improve co-operation in teams (Lazear 2000, p. 626). Gibbs and Levinson (2000) argue that economics has little to say about the internal workings of

[1] Team production may also involve individual compensation, but where the actions of agents are complementary and a higher level of one action raises the marginal product of other actions.

teams, and refer to the management literature that emphasizes learning, job enrichment, information sharing and collaboration.

The use of teams in health care has recently been reviewed by Ratto *et al.* (2001). They argue that the main issue within the NHS is how to define the team prior to the introduction of team-based compensation. Medical group partnerships have been analysed in the context of teams. There is an incentive for partners to shirk and free ride on the effort of others if revenues are shared amongst partners, or where joint output is the only indicator of inputs. Although such a system spreads risks, it reduces efficiency. If the compensation of an individual physician is directly linked to output (and therefore effort), there will be incentives to be efficient, but risk is not shared. Crucial to these models has therefore been the extent that risk aversion is a determinant of internal compensation method and of the behaviour (effort) of physicians.

For example, Gaynor and Gertler (1995) examined the relationship between the degree of risk sharing, compensation and effort in primary care physicians in the USA in medical group practice. They specify a model where demand is uncertain, and where physicians choose 'effort' to maximize utility in response to the incentives in the firm's compensation structure. The utility-maximizing level of effort is where the marginal revenue product of effort is equal to its marginal disutility. They go on to derive comparative static results of the effect of changes in internal compensation on the number of patients seen (defined as 'effort'). They also examine the effect of risk aversion on choice of compensation structure. Increased risk aversion leads to compensation methods that are more likely to involve the sharing of rewards. Compensation schemes that are more closely linked to output have a large and positive effect on output, measured in terms of patient visits.

Bradford (1995) suggested that malpractice risk helped to explain the formation of medical partnerships. He argued that when risk premia are paid by the group and shared equally amongst partners, then increased malpractice risk will reduce individual effort. This will lead to increased administrative costs within a partnership to increase effort, thus placing partnerships at a competitive disadvantage. Therefore partnerships become less probable as malpractice risk increases. The predictions were rejected for primary care but confirmed for surgical specialities where the financial consequences of being sued are much greater.

Encinosa *et al.* (1997) examined why compensation may not always be linked to productivity in medical groups, using the sociological concept of 'group norms' incorporated into an economic framework of risk sharing and multitasking. Group norms are defined as the social interactions resulting from comparisons of effort and pay within groups. They demonstrate that group income and effort norms make small groups more likely to adopt equal sharing rules than large groups, and that risk aversion and multitasking make equal sharing more likely in large groups. Using the same data set as Gaynor and Gertler (1995), they find evidence that group norms do influence choice of compensation method, in addition to the usual factors analysed in principal–agent models (risk aversion and multitasking).

BUREAUCRATIC RULES

The problems of multitasking and subjective performance evaluation may lead firms to reward performance based on bureaucratic rules that remove the element of discretion and are less likely to be related to measured performance (Prendergast 1999). They may construct rules to govern the behaviour of agents where there are multiple tasks and multiple principals (Wilson 1989). These rules can be efficient but they can also lead to distortion of effort where the agents themselves or their representatives (trade unions) are involved in their construction. Rules that limit the discretion of middle-ranking agents/principals may also reduce 'currying favour' in hierarchical agencies. Such rules for example may require that the agent spend a fixed amount of time on a specific task. The existence of such rules results in the 'micromanagement' of agents, especially where there are multiple tasks and multiple principals. Micromanagement may therefore be an efficient way of dealing with the multiplicity of outcomes and principals. For example, the payment of automatic annual increments to salary is such a rule, as well as maxima and minima in pay scales. There may also be minimum experience requirements where workers must stay in a particular position before promotion, regardless of performance or ability. Another example is the weight given to seniority in promotion and layoff decisions. This would be efficient if seniority is related to ability and performance, but this may not always be the case. These rules may also be efficient if they reduce the likelihood that workers will 'curry favour' with their supervisors (Milgrom & Roberts 1988).

Bureaucratic rules are an element of many reward systems in health care, particularly for salaried payment where annual automatic advancement along a salary scale is unrelated to performance or any type of subjective evaluation. There may also be similar rules where promotion may not occur until an individual has reached a minimum level of experience in a job, again regardless of their ability. In the UK, GPs receive a fixed payment for being senior, defined in terms of a minimum level of experience. These rules are explicit and apply to everyone, so they may avoid some of the problems of subjective performance evaluation. In the absence of direct measures of performance or where measurement of performance is costly, employers may judge that the basis of these rules is an adequate proxy for performance and would therefore be efficient.

In the case of the UK NHS, there is tension between the autonomy of the local decision-maker and the desire for the centre to retain some control over their actions. Guidelines, guidance, policy documents, regulations, advice and laws are regularly issued and the complex and multitasking nature of the industry means that the focus is often on the process and inputs rather than outcomes. Furthermore, the objectives of local decision-makers and subsequent activities may not be consistent with national objectives of geographical/regional equity, which increases the likelihood of central intervention.

INTERNAL AND EXTERNAL MARKETS AS INDUCERS OF EFFORT

The focus in health economics on the role of explicit incentives in the context of principal–agent models has meant that other types of implicit incentives have been ignored in the literature. In particular, it is important to explain why effort is expended by health professionals in the absence of any formal explicit incentive schemes, for example where salary payment is used. It has already been suggested that ethical concerns will play a role in inducing effort in health care, but there are other factors that are likely to be important and that can be altered by principals. These are incentives in promotions, career concerns and efficiency wages. Each is discussed below.

INCENTIVES IN PROMOTIONS

In the UK hospital sector, doctors, nurses, managers and other workers in the NHS are paid by salary which is linked to a job hierarchy, promotions and bonus schemes. More generally, it should be recognized that this is a more common way of providing incentives than pay for performance (Prendergast 1999). Theoretical models in this area use tournament theory, where a group of agents compete for a fixed set of prizes (Lazear & Rosen 1981). In this theory, individuals are motivated by comparison with peers or a standard, where performance is defined by winning a 'prize' (e.g. a promotion or bonus). A prediction of this theory is that greater prizes lead to more effort, and this has been confirmed empirically in the area of sport (see Prendergast 1999 for a review of this literature). This provides further evidence that incentives matter. A further prediction is that in the case of a single prize, to motivate efficient behaviour, the prize must increase with the number of competitors. The theory also predicts that in a 'biased tournament', where one agent has a better chance of winning, an agent who is behind may reduce effort and be more likely to engage in risky behaviours. Tournaments are, however, competitive and so agents are unlikely to help each other when incentives are strong. This is especially the case when there is a large spread between the wages of a promotion hierarchy. It follows that firms may choose a more compressed wage structure if a co-operative work environment is important – this is relevant in teams but also in the public sector where more compressed wage structures are observed due to the central negotiation of pay (Lazear 2000). A dynamic perspective introduces issues concerned with workers progressing through a firm's hierarchy, and how this is related to the returns to promotion. The existence of convex wage structures, where the returns to promotion increase as a worker moves up the hierarchy, has been the subject of theoretical and empirical analysis. The slope of the wage structure can be explained by income effects, where it takes more money to induce effort from high-paid workers compared to low-paid workers. There may also be more effort required in a senior job, so that the marginal return to effort is positively associated with rank. Convex wage schedules may also offer rents to senior workers as a means of providing incentives to all workers (Rosen 1986). Part of the return from getting promoted may be the increased probability of getting promoted again in the future – the 'option value' of promotion. This is also relevant to 'career concerns' discussed below. This raises issues such as 'fast track' promotions, serial correlation in wage increases and promotion rates, and the relationship between promotions and exits (Baker *et al.* 1994b; Gibbons 1997). It is also important to relate wage growth (or the chance of a promotion) to firm or worker effects, if firm-level incentives are to be used to improve effort. The empirical literature also examines the extent to which promotions come from the upper deciles of the wage distribution of lower grades, and the destination of promotees in the wage distribution of the higher-grade job.

Incentives in promotions are relevant in health care where salaried payment schedules define a hierarchy of pay scales, and also where bonuses and promotion are based on competition. For example, the post of NHS consultant can be thought of as a 'prize', that not only brings with it higher remuneration (and the opportunity for further bonuses through distinction awards and opportunities to work in the private sector), but also substantial non-pecuniary aspects to the 'prize' that create incentives for effort, such as reputation and status, clinical responsibility and autonomy. This creates strong incentives for effort from more junior doctors, as evidenced by their very long hours of work. One potential effect of altering the contract of employment for NHS consultants ('the prize') may be that it will change the effort of more junior doctors, but this will depend on how the size of the prize changes.

The theory also predicts that the strong competitive incentives may mean that co-operation and teamwork between hospital doctors may be more limited than where the incentives from promotion were less strong. This is likely to be the case where there is a large spread of earnings in a promotion hierarchy, as between junior doctors and consultants who hold distinction awards. Hospital doctors who have different career and work–leisure preferences can opt to become 'staff grade' doctors rather than consultants. This group of doctors are often regarded as 'failed' consultants who have not got the ability to be consultants. However, a proportion of these will select themselves out of the competition for reasons related to work–leisure preferences. This is evidence of the operation of 'up or out' rules that have been identified in the theoretical literature.

In contrast, self-employed GPs in the UK have no such promotion or career structure and so would be expected to have weaker incentives for effort than if such a structure existed. The introduction of a career structure for GPs may therefore increase effort and productivity, although these effects may be traded off against the weaker incentives for effort in a salary system compared to the current mixed system of payment.

Tournaments also apply to hospitals in England, whereby the top performers are rewarded by financial means, in the form of access to a 'performance fund', and also by non-financial means, where hospitals will be given greater autonomy. Given that there is no clear distribution of residual rights or property rights in health care organizations in the UK, such financial rewards will not be directly related to managers' pay, but rather to access to resources for the hospital. Therefore, the extent to which such tournaments will provide sufficient incentive to change behaviour is open to question. If the decision-makers are driven by financial incentives then only by tying in hospital performance with chief executives' remuneration will they be motivated to respond to these indicators. More likely, the hospital manager has a more complex utility function that includes arguments such as status and prestige.

CAREER CONCERNS

The role of the external labour market is also important in providing incentives for effort through career concerns. It is argued that the external market acts in this way when good performance by the worker in current employment improves future employment prospects (Fama 1980). Effort can therefore occur without explicit pay for performance contracts. This emphasizes the role of reputation: incentives are provided by the external labour market when the worker's current performance influences the market's belief about the worker's ability, and so influences the worker's future compensation. Outside contractual options matter in the provision of incentives for effort. However, these incentives alone may produce an inefficient pattern of effort over time if workers work too hard in the early years to establish their reputation, and not hard enough in later years once their reputation has been established (Gibbons & Murphy 1992). Effort levels will therefore fall over time, and so contracts may need to become more explicit by the use of pay for performance measures as tenure increases. It also follows that current performance may need to be more closely linked to rewards and penalties for workers with short tenure, rather than for those with longer tenure. Career concerns can also induce myopia, where agents care too much about short-term returns.

EFFICIENCY WAGES

Efficiency wages refers to a situation in which wages are not linked to current output but firms overpay workers to induce effort and the additional cost of job loss to the worker leads to an efficient level of effort (Shapiro & Stiglitz 1984; Malcolmson 1999). There is a large labour economics literature in this area with conflicting results and explanations as to the reasons for and effects of these wage premia (Prendergast 1999). For example, if turnover costs to the employer are high then higher wages may be offered to reduce turnover rather than increase effort (Malcolmson 1999). However, wages above the apparent market clearing level may also be explained by the presence of unobserved job characteristics or abilities of workers. Hence the existence and motivational effect of efficiency wages has not been conclusively demonstrated.

Related to this is deferred compensation, where workers are overpaid when old and underpaid when young, relative to their marginal product – wages rise more rapidly than marginal product (Lazear 1979). One explanation for this empirical observation is that it encourages workers to stay, so reducing the costs of turnover. It may also reflect workers' own preferences for wages over the lifecycle. A more common explanation is that older workers are paid rents to encourage extra effort, but this is also attractive to younger workers who may be more likely to stay in the firm long enough to attain those rents. Younger workers can then be offered lower compensation while maintaining incentives (Akerlof & Katz 1989).

Compensation is not therefore necessarily related to productivity, and so deferred compensation may be more prevalent in firms where productivity is difficult to measure. The incentives of deferred compensation may also be an explanation for the importance given to seniority in pay, promotion and recruitment and retention decisions, independent of productivity concerns.

Lazear (2000) examines the threat of dismissal as providing incentives for effort under such a scheme. A minimum standard exists and if effort falls below this, the worker is dismissed. If the employer wants to increase effort the minimum standard is increased. However, if workers are heterogeneous then a common minimum standard may lead to inefficiencies as low-ability workers are forced to work harder than is optimal, and high-ability workers put in less effort than is optimal.

This has implications for the pay of senior NHS managers. Chief executives of Hospital Trusts have poor job security relative to other public sector employees. This may act as a disciplinary device on senior management's performance. However, in order to attract good managers into the service, in accordance with the standard compensating differences argument, compensatingly high salaries are required. However, chief executive salary levels in the NHS are below the equivalent private sector levels (News Focus 2001).

MOTIVATION, SOCIAL CONTEXT AND NON-FINANCIAL INCENTIVES

In health care, it has long been recognized that health professionals are likely to have the patient's utility (or at least health status) as an argument in their utility functions. Nevertheless, the role of incentives in influencing the trade-off between patients' interests and other arguments in health professionals' utility functions has not yet been explored empirically. The source of the motivation of self-interested individuals in economic theory is financial. Agency theory (and labour economics more generally) focuses entirely on the role of wages and remuneration and of associated relative price effects as influencing behaviour when other factors are held constant. Fehr and Falk (2002) argue that, 'this narrow view of human motivation may severely limit progress in understanding incentives.'

Sociologists and psychologists emphasize the social context of reward and penalties and the non-pecuniary sources of motivation. This literature is being recognized by some economists as relevant and is being incorporated into further developments of theory, although empirical work has not yet caught up (Kreps 1997; Prendergast 1999; Dixit 2001). Two aspects of this literature are relevant in health care: intrinsic motivation and social context.

INTRINSIC MOTIVATION

Contrary to the assumption in economics that workers experience disutility from working, many individuals obtain positive but diminishing marginal utility from working, although the precise nature of this relationship will differ across jobs. The reason for positive utility from working is job satisfaction and intrinsic motivation. The latter is defined as when a task is undertaken and no reward is received except the task itself. The classic example is the voluntary donation of blood (Titmuss 1970). Gibbs and Levinson (2000) relate intrinsic motivation to job design, and outline the Hackman–Oldman model that shows how job enrichment, adding complexity or more tasks, generates intrinsic motivation and increases productivity. The meaningfulness of work, responsibility for outcomes, and knowledge of the impact of outcomes all increase intrinsic work motivation in this model. Gibbs and Levinson define intrinsic motivation as aspects of job design that affect the marginal disutility of effort, particularly the issues of learning new tasks and the intellectual aspects of work. This also emphasizes the ability of individuals to show initiative and have autonomy.

In addition to tasks being interesting, Frey (1997) argues that intrinsic motivation will be high where personal relationships exist between principals and agents that imply recognition, trust and loyalty. Additionally, the agent's participation in higher-level decision-making may foster intrinsic motivation, compared to hierarchical decision-making.

Intrinsic motivation is also likely to be present in professional groups or where a 'public service' ethos exists. The existence of a public service ethos has been discussed in empirical work that sought to explain the wage differences between public and private sector workers. The 'public service ethos' can be linked back to career concerns and implicit incentives for effort where there are group-level rules of behaviour and conduct, or where there are strong ethical and moral responsibilities encompassed in jobs (Dewatripont *et al.* 1999; Dixit 2001).

However, Frey (1997) outlines more fundamental concerns with respect to the relationship between extrinsic motivation and intrinsic motivation. Drawing upon theory and evidence from cognitive social psychology, he argues that there may be cases where extrinsic incentives 'crowd out' intrinsic motivation (Motivation Crowding Theory). This is where the introduction of external monetary rewards, where previously there were none, can undermine intrinsic motivation, ' . . . and even reverse the most fundamental economic law, namely that raising monetary incentives increases supply' (Frey & Jegen 2001). Frey and Jegen argue that for tasks where intrinsic motivation is high, the introduction of extrinsic rewards may be inefficient and lead to lower productivity and participation – paying for performance may demotivate workers. The external intervention may reduce the agent's marginal benefit from performing the task, and this can dominate the relative price effect. A body of empirical evidence exists to support motivation crowding theory (Frey & Jegen 2001).

Extrinsic incentives can also be viewed as controlling, and may reduce trust, including when extrinsic intervention is in the form of monitoring (Frey 1993). This is one explanation why explicit performance contracts are not used more extensively.

The role of intrinsic motivation in health care may be particularly strong where health professionals have strong ethical concerns and where patients' welfare is an argument in their own utility function (Jones 2002). High intrinsic motivation may be more likely for those in direct contact with patients, rather than for managers and administrators. The key question is the effect of extrinsic financial incentives or monitoring on productivity and effort. It is important to examine situations where an extrinsic incentive is introduced where previously there was no financial incentive and high intrinsic motivation for a task. However, this issue has not been examined empirically in health care, although some commentators have suggested that intrinsic motivation in the medical profession may be declining (Jones 2002).

Intrinsic motivation, and the trust which it may engender, could be explanations (in addition to the problems associated with multitasking and asymmetry of information) for the general absence of pay and performance systems in the UK NHS. Intrinsic motivation may have negated (or be perceived to have negated) the need for routine monitoring systems, especially when balanced against the transactions costs of monitoring.

SOCIAL CONTEXT

Social comparison theory is based in social psychology, but has been used by economists (Frank 1985) to explain that behaviour is motivated by comparisons with peers and that individuals obtain utility from such comparisons, e.g. from relative levels of income. Wage distributions will then be compressed since workers at the bottom need to be compensated to be there and workers at the top will 'pay' to be there. Issues about social context are also important in team working, where social disapproval, adherence to group norms and reciprocity may be important determinants of behaviour. These issues highlight the role of equity and equality in the workplace. The evidence for the existence of these motivations is reviewed by Fehr and Falk (2002). Their role in health care may be particularly important to investigate further.

The broader social and institutional context of financial incentives in health care has been examined by Giacomini et al. (1996). A conceptual framework is presented that views financial incentives as a function of individuals' and organizations' perceptions of the associated change in funding. The incentive properties (i.e. behavioural effects) of a funding change are not necessarily embodied in the funding change, and depend on how the funding change is communicated and perceived in the policy environment (Giacomini & Goldsmith 1996; Giacomini et al. 1996). Funding changes therefore carry messages that are open to some interpretation, with this interpretation dependent on the social and institutional context of key stakeholders. The behavioural effect can therefore deviate from what the policy-maker intended.

DISCUSSION

Several developments in the economic theory of incentives and how they apply in health care have been reviewed in this chapter. It is argued that there are many aspects of this theory that have not yet been examined by economists in general and health economists in particular. Some key developments in the psychology and sociology literature that are relevant in examining the effectiveness of incentives schemes have also been reviewed briefly. Several messages emerge for research and policy in the area of incentives in health care.

There is ample evidence from within health care and from the broader economics literature that explicit pay for performance does influence behaviour, but will be efficient only for simple jobs. In complex jobs and where output is difficult to define and measure, paying for performance may lead to inefficiency through a focus on the measured performance, rather than on other valuable aspects of activity. The role of mixed or 'blended' systems of payment is important here in reducing the worst effects of each specific payment method (Robinson 2001). Although this conclusion is perhaps not new to health economists, it is important to reiterate this message to policy-makers who continue to experiment with 'pay for performance' in health care. Further research into the effects of changes in these systems is valuable in determining which 'mix' of payment methods is congruent with the objectives of patients and the health care system.

It is important to recognize that incentives for effort can exist in the absence of explicit pay for performance contracts through incentives in promotions, career concerns, subjective performance evaluation, intrinsic motivation and social context. Promotions would appear to play an important role in certain parts of the UK health service. For example, although salary payment is often regarded as providing few incentives for effort, most employees in the public sector are salaried and exert effort (including academics). Hospital consultants, nurses and some GPs are paid by salary in the UK NHS. The key question is whether these systems are optimal and how they can be changed at the margin to promote greater efficiency and equity. The design of salary scales and career structures has not traditionally been the realm of health economists, yet they seem crucial as a tool to change incentives and alter behaviour. Continuing changes to the contracts of GPs, hospital consultants and other health professionals in the UK should be examined in this light. Research is required on the promotion and career structures of health care professionals to examine the relationship between changes in rank with changes in wages, productivity and employer and employee characteristics.

The role of subjective assessment of performance is important in many contexts in health care. In the UK, this is the main method by which the performance of hospitals is being assessed, although many quantitative performance indicators also inform this. The introduction of annual performance appraisal for GPs and hospital consultants is relevant here. Instances where subjective performance evaluation replaces the use of objective performance measures (and vice versa) seem an important area of empirical research and the net effect on efficiency is not known.

Mooney and Ryan (1993) suggested more research is needed into the utility functions of health care providers and consumers before incentives and regulation can be designed to enhance efficiency. Although there is some evidence of such research being conducted, there is much still to explore (Ryan *et al.* 2001; Scott 2001). The assumption, used in most principal–agent models, that monetary factors are the only component of the utility functions of providers is untenable in the health care (and other) contexts. The role of intrinsic motivation and strong ethical concerns may reduce the need for strong explicit performance contracts in many areas of health care, although there is still a need to alter performance at the margin. Where strong extrinsic incentives exist (e.g. physicians in HMOs in the USA), intrinsic motivation may be reduced and physicians may obtain greater utility from the extrinsic reward than from the task itself. Of course, the nature of intrinsic motivation needs to be examined: doctors or managers may be ethically or intrinsically motivated but that will not necessarily take the health care sector in the direction that other stakeholders want.

The need to examine the utility functions of providers is still an important area of further work. Studies that examine the relative impact of financial vs. non-financial means to change behaviour in specific contexts are particularly important. For example, the focus of the implementation of evidence-based medicine is on changing physician behaviour through the use of educational interventions (Bero *et al.* 1998; Mason *et al.* 2001). These strategies operate by reducing information costs for doctors, and changing their perceptions of the costs and benefits of their own actions. However, this needs to be compared to the effects of using financial incentives to encourage or discourage specific interventions. This is a key area of research.

There are a number of issues that this chapter has not addressed in detail, but which are nevertheless important. These are the development of theoretical models, the measurement of productivity in health care (in terms of what outcomes patients and society values), and the measurement and analysis of subjective phenomena.

In addition to the above, there are several key issues that require further empirical research. The first is the analysis of health care personnel data sets to examine incentives in careers and promotions. This is an untapped area that could provide new insights into the role of incentives in changing the behaviour of health professionals where salaried payment dominates, such as in the UK NHS. It will also be important for health economics to make progess in researching the non-pecuniary motivations that are amenable to policy change, as well as examining more carefully the role of social and institutional context in influencing behaviour. The interactions between economics and psychology and sociology need to be explored here. This research is necessary if answers are to be provided to the policy questions of how to change the behaviour of health professionals to improve efficiency and equity in health care.

ACKNOWLEDGEMENTS

The authors would like to thank Sally Stearns, Robert Elliott, Alan Maynard and participants of the HERU workshop for comments on earlier versions. The Health Economics Research Unit is funded by the Chief Scientist Office of the Scottish Executive Health Department. The views are those of the authors and not the funders.

REFERENCES

Akerlof G and Katz L (1989) Workers trust funds and the logic of wage profiles. *Quarterly Journal of Economics*, **104**, 525–536.

Baker G (1992) Incentive contracts and performance measurement. *Journal of Political Economy*, **43**, 598–614.

Baker G, Gibbons R and Murphy KJ (1994a) Subjective performance measures in optimal incentive contracts. *Quarterly Journal of Economics*, **109**, 1125–1156.

Baker G, Gibbs M and Holmstrom B (1994b) The internal economics of the firm: evidence from personnel data. *Quarterly Journal of Economics*, **109**, 881–919.

Bero LA, Grilli R, Grimshaw JM, Harvey E, Oxman AD and Thomson A (1998) Closing the gap between research and practice: an overview of systematic reviews of interventions to promote the implementation of research findings. *British Medical Journal*, **317**, 465–468.

Bloor K and Maynard A (1992) *Rewarding excellence? Consultants' distinction awards and the need for reform*. Discussion Paper 100, Centre for Health Economics, University of York.

Bradford WD (1995) Solo versus group practice in the medical profession. The influence of malpractice risk. *Health Economics*, **4**, 95–112.

Burgess S and Metcalfe P (1999a) *Incentives in organisations: a selective overview of the literature with application to the public sector*. Working Paper 99/016, Centre for Market and Public Organisation, University of Bristol.

Burgess S and Metcalfe P (1999b) *The use of incentive schemes in the public and private sectors: evidence from British establishments*. Working Paper 00/15, Centre for Market and Public Organisation, University of Bristol.

Chalkley M and Malcolmson JM (1998) Contracting for health services when patient demand does not reflect quality. *Journal of Health Economics*, **17**, 1–19.

Dewatripoint M, Jewitt I and Tirole J (1999) The economics of career concerns. Part I. Comparing information structures. *Review of Economic Studies*, **66**, 183–198.

Dixit A (2001) *Incentives and organisations in the public sector: an interpretative review*. Paper presented at 'Incentives in the Public Sector' workshop, Centre for Market and Public Organisation, University of Bristol.

Encinosa WE, Gaynor M and Rebitzer JB (1997) *The sociology of groups and the economics of incentives: theory and evidence on compensation systems*. Working Paper 5953, National Bureau of Economic Research Cambridge, MA.

Fama E (1980) Agency problems and the theory of the firm. *Journal of Political Economy*, **88**, 288–307.

Fehr E and Falk A (2002) Psychological foundations of incentives. *European Economic Review*, **46**, 687–724.

Frank R (1985) *Choosing the Right Pond: Human Behaviour and the Quest for Status.* Oxford University Press, New York.

Frey BS (1993) Does monitoring increase work effort? The rivalry with trust and loyalty. *Economic Inquiry*, **31**, 663–670.

Frey BS (1997) Not just for the money. *An Economic Theory of Personal Motivation.* Edward Elgar, Cheltenham.

Frey BS and Jegen R (2001) Motivation crowding theory: a survey of empirical evidence. *Journal of Economic Surveys*, **15**, 589–611.

Gaynor M and Gertler P (1995) Moral hazard and risk spreading in partnerships. *Rand Journal of Economics*, **26**, 591–613.

Giacomini M and Goldsmith L (1996) *Case study methodology for studying financial incentives in context.* Working Paper 96-15, McMaster University Centre for Health Economics and Policy Analysis.

Giacomini M, Hurley J, Lomas J, Bhatia V and Goldsmith L (1996) *The many meanings of money: a health policy analysis framework for understanding financial incentives in context.* Working Paper 96-6, McMaster University Centre for Health Economics and Policy Analysis.

Gibbons R (1997) Incentives and careers in organisations. In D Kreps and K Wallis (Eds), *Advances in Economics and Econometrics: Theory and Applications.* Cambridge University Press, Cambridge.

Gibbons R and Murphy KJ (1992) Optimal incentive contracts in the presence of career concerns: theory and evidence. *Journal of Political Economy*, **100**, 468–505.

Gibbons R and Waldman M (1999) Careers in organisations: theory and evidence. In O Ashenfelter and D Card (Eds), *Handbook of Labour Economics, Volume 3.* Elsevier, Amsterdam.

Gibbs M and Levinson A (2000) *The economic approach to personnel research.* Paper presented at the Society for the Advancement of Behavioural Economics.

Goddard M, Mannion R and Smith P (2000) Enhancing performance in health care: a theoretical perspective on agency and the role of information. *Health Economics*, **9**, 95–107.

Gosden T, Forland F, Kristiansen IS, Sutton M, Leese B, Guiffrida A, Sergison M and Pedersen L (2001) Impact of payment method on the behaviour of primary care physicians: a systematic review. *Journal of Health Services Research and Policy*, **6**, 44–55.

Guiffrida A, Gosden T, Forland F, Kristiansen IS, Sergison M, Leese B, Pedersen L and Sutton M (2001) Target payments in primary care: effects on professional practice and health care outcomes (Cochrane Review). In *The Cochrane Library, Issue 2.* Update Software, Oxford.

Hansen D (1997) Worker performance and group incentives: a case study. *Industrial Labour Relations Review*, **51**, 37–49.

Hausman D and LeGrand J (1999) Incentives in health policy: primary and secondary care in the British National Health Service. *Social Science and Medicine*, **49**, 1299–1307.

Hellinger FJ (1996) The impact of financial incentives on physician behaviour in managed care plans: a review of the evidence. *Medical Care Research Review*, **53**, 294–314.

Holmstrom B and Milgrom P (1991) Multitask principal–agent analyses: incentive contracts, asset ownership and job design. *Journal of Law, Economics and Organisation*, **7**, 24–52.

Hughes D and Yule B (1992) The effect of per item fees on the behaviour of general practitioners. *Journal of Health Economics*, **4**, 413–438.

Jones R (2002) Declining altruism in medicine. *British Medical Journal*, **324**, 624–625.

Kreps DM (1997) Intrinsic motivation and extrinsic incentives. *American Economic Review*, **87**, 359–364.

Labelle R, Stoddart G and Rice T (1994) A re-examination of the meaning and importance of supplier induced demand. *Journal of Health Economics*, **13**, 347–368.

Lazear E (1979) Why is there mandatory retirement? *Journal of Political Economy*, **87**, 1261–1284.

Lazear E (1999) *Personnel economics: past lessons and future directions*. Working Paper 6957, National Bureau of Economic Research, Cambridge, MA.

Lazear E (2000) The future of personnel economics. *The Economic Journal*, **110**, 611–639.

Lazear E and Rosen S (1981) Rank order tournaments as optimal labour contracts. *Journal of Political Economy*, **89**, 841–864.

Malcolmson JM (1999) Individual employment contracts. In O Ashenfelter and D Card (Eds), *Handbook of Labour Economics, Volume 3*. Elsevier, Amsterdam.

Mason J, Freemantle N, Nazereth I, Eccles M, Haines A and Drummond M (2001) When is it cost-effective to change the behaviour of health professionals? *Journal of the American Medical Association*, **286**, 2988–2992.

McGuire T (2000) Physician agency. In AJ Culyer and JP Newhouse (Eds), *Handbook of Health Economics, Volume 1A*. Elsevier, Amsterdam.

Milgrom P and Roberts J (1988) An economic approach to influence in organisations. *American Journal of Sociology*, **94**, 154–179.

Mooney G and Ryan M (1993) Agency in health care: getting beyond first principles. *Journal of Health Economics*, **12**, 125–238.

News Focus (2001) The price is right? *Health Service Journal*.

O'Cathain A, Brazier JE, Milner PC and Fall M (1992) Cost effectiveness of minor surgery in general practice: a prospective comparison with hospital practice. *British Journal of General Practice*, **42**, 13–17.

Prendergast C (1999) The provision of incentives in firms. *Journal of Economic Literature*, **37**, 7–63.

Preyra C and Pink G (2001) Balancing incentives in the compensation contract of non-profit hospital CEOs. *Journal of Health Economics*, **20**, 509–525.

Propper C (1995) Agency and incentives in the NHS internal market. *Social Science and Medicine*, **40**, 1683–1690.

Ratto M, Burgess S, Croxson B, Jewitt I and Propper C (2001) *Team-based incentives in the NHS: an economic analysis*. Working Paper 01/37, Centre for Market and Public Organisation, University of Bristol.

Rice T (2001) *The Economics of Health Reconsidered*. Health Administration Press, Chicago.

Robinson JC (2001) Theory and practice in the design of physician payment incentives. *Milbank Quarterly*, **79**, 149–177.

Rosen S (1986) Prizes and incentives in elimination tournaments. *American Economic Review*, **76**, 921–939.

Ryan M, Scott DA, Bate A, van Teijlingen E, Russell EM, Napper M, Reeves C and Robb C (2001) Eliciting public preferences for health care: a systematic review and evaluation of methods. *Health Technology Assessment*, **5**(5).

Scott A (2001) *Agency and incentives in general practice*. PhD Thesis, University of Aberdeen.

Scott A and Vick S (1999) Patients, doctors and contracts: an application of principal–agent theory to the doctor–patient relationship. *Scottish Journal of Political Economy*, **46**, 111–134.

Shapiro C and Stiglitz J (1984) Equilibrium unemployment as a discipline device. *American Economic Review*, **74**, 433–444.

Sloan FA (2000) Not-for-profit ownership and hospital behaviour. In AJ Culyer and JP Newhouse (Eds), *Handbook of Health Economics*. North-Holland, Amsterdam.

Titmuss RM (1970) *The Gift Relationship*. Allen and Unwin, London.

Vick S and Scott A (1998) Agency in health care. Examining patients' preferences for attributes of the doctor–patient relationship. *Journal of Health Economics*, **17**, 587–606.

Weiss A (1987) Incentives and worker behaviour. In H Nalbantian (Ed.), *Information, Incentives and Risk Sharing*. Rowan and Littlefield, New Jersey.

Whynes D (1993) Can performance monitoring solve the public services' principal agent problem? *Scottish Journal of Political Economy*, **40**(4), 434–446.

Wilson JQ (1989) *Bureaucracy: What Government Agencies Do and Why they Do it*. Basic Books, New York.

6

The Nursing Labour Market

ROBERT ELLIOTT
Health Economics Research Unit, University of Aberdeen

DIANE SKÅTUN
Health Economics Research Unit, University of Aberdeen

EMANUELA ANTONAZZO
Department of Economics, University of Bologna and Regional Health Agency of
Emilia Romagna

INTRODUCTION

There were over half a million nurses working in the UK at the end of the
twentieth century. Over 90% of nurses are women and nursing is the largest
source of professional employment for women in the UK. 11% of women
working in Scotland and 8.6% of women working in England work in the
National Health Service (NHS) and the majority of these work as nurses
(Elliott et al. 2002). In 1990 6.3% of all female nurses and 14.7% of all male
nurses working in the NHS came from ethnic minorities. Both these
percentages were much larger than their respective percentages in the
workforce as a whole (Shields & Price 2002). Nursing is different in important
respects from most other jobs. Nurses enjoy very high levels of public esteem
and the task of nursing has frequently been described as more of a vocation
than a job.

A substantial number of nurses are employed in the private sector. They
comprise perhaps as much as 10% of the total nursing workforce (Elliott et al.
2002), but they are concentrated in London and the South of England.
Scotland employs more nurses per head of population than England: it had 10
nurses per 1000 population in 1999 compared to 6.8 per 1000 in England in
that same year.

Advances in Health Economics. Edited by Anthony Scott, Alan Maynard and Robert Elliott.
© 2003 John Wiley & Sons, Ltd

Nurses constituted 45% of the total staff in the NHS and their salary bill accounted for almost 50% of the total NHS salary bill in 1998 (Office of Health Economics 1999). In 2000 the total pay bill for nurses was around £8 billion, or between 2 and 3% of total public expenditure (Health Departments for Great Britain 2001). Most recently the Wanless Report (2002) has suggested that the UK may need to employ over 100,000 additional nurses over the next 20 years if it is to provide a high-quality health service by 2022. The recent endorsement of this report by the government and its decision to increase spending on health care by almost 50% over the next five years suggests that the demand for nurses will grow strongly over this period. Attracting appropriate numbers into the nursing profession will be a key to realizing the goal of providing a world-class health care system.

Discussion about the nursing labour market in the UK has recently focused on recruitment and retention issues. There have been severe shortages of nurses in some areas of the UK, principally London and the South East, and in some specializations. Recent policies, in England in particular, have sought to increase the numbers in training, while increasing recruitment from other countries. Some hospital trusts in England have introduced 'golden hellos', lump sum cash payments, for those returning to NHS employment, others have sought to recruit nurses from abroad. Also in England some NHS Trusts have introduced flexible working arrangements, childcare support and housing subsidies in an attempt to increase retention and recruitment.

Underpinning the discussion of these issues has been concerns over the relative pay of nurses and the general attractiveness of nursing as a career. Attempts are being made to 'modernize' the pay system by introducing greater regional and grade flexibility (Health Departments for Great Britain 2001). Yet in Scotland the position seems to be very different: recruitment problems, except in some specialist areas, are far less severe than in England. Indeed vacancy rates for nurses fell during the late 1990s at a time when they were rising in the rest of the Scottish economy.

Nursing shortages can be addressed from both the demand and supply sides. The demand for nurses depends upon the size of the NHS budget and the organization and allocation of labour within the NHS. Whatever the size of the budget for health care services the distribution of these resources between doctors, nurses and auxiliary employees is critical and this division of labour will have important consequences for the demand for nurses on two fronts. The introduction of more advanced clinical roles for nurses means that they can now be regarded as potential substitutes for some roles that have traditionally been filled by doctors. While at the other end of the skill spectrum, there is the potential to substitute some of the more traditional nursing roles by auxiliary staff. However any change in the organizational structure and specification of the job of nursing will also affect the attractiveness of nursing as a career and thus have supply-side effects.

In this chapter the existing economic research into the labour market for nurses in the UK will be reviewed. The way in which economists model, in an attempt to understand, the determinants of the supply of labour to nursing will be explored and the available empirical evidence of labour supply will be reviewed. Other indicators of labour market supply resulting from attempts to directly measure job satisfaction will also be examined and research into the pay of nurses and the determinants of the demand for nurses analysed. The research issues arising from this literature are summarized.

LONG-RUN EQUILIBRIUM IN THE MARKET

The theory of compensating differentials has been described as 'the fundamental (long-run) market equilibrium construct in labour economics' (Rosen 1986). It originates in the writings of Adam Smith who wrote in *The Wealth of Nations* that 'the whole of the advantages and disadvantages of different employments of labour and stock must, in the same neighbourhood be either perfectly equal or continually leading to equality. If in the same neighbourhood there was any employment either evidently more or less advantageous than the rest, so many people would crowd into it in the one case, and so many would desert it in the other, that its advantages would soon return to the level of other employment' (Smith 1776). The forces of competition would equalize the net advantages associated with different jobs.

According to Smith the net advantages of jobs could be described in terms of five different sets of characteristics of jobs. First the 'agreeableness' of the job, today we would term this the nature of the working environment. Second the 'cost of learning the business', today we talk of the magnitude and dimensions of the human capital investment required for a particular job. The third according to Smith was the constancy of employment, in today's terms the security of the job. The remaining two were termed the trust to be reposed and the probability of success and describe respectively jobs in which honesty is required and in which there is a high variance in wages.

According to Smith these characteristics of jobs determined their attractiveness and therefore as Smith's statement above reveals, the supply of labour to different jobs. The theory is essentially a theory of the determinants of long-run labour supply. The statement is silent on demand conditions in the labour market. It takes labour demand and technology as given and looks at the response of labour supply to these. The theory provides the framework for evaluating the empirical work on labour supply. It informs us that the determinants of the supply of labour to nursing and other jobs will be the education and training required to do the job, the level and predictability of pay, and the many other non-pecuniary aspects of the job, such as the safety and pleasantness of the working environment. How many of these dimensions are captured in the empirical work we shall evaluate?

EMPIRICAL METHOD OF LABOUR SUPPLY ANALYSIS

Nursing labour supply represents a specific case of the more general theory of labour supply. It combines a number of dimensions which distinguish it from the general theory appropriate to describe labour supply to other markets. First the vast majority of labour supplied to this occupation is by women. Second, in the UK at least, a very large proportion of women undertake a substantial amount of non-market work within the household, caring for other members of the household. This introduces a distinct dimension as well as a life-cycle pattern into the labour supply of nurses and many other women. Third, nurses appear to exhibit stronger preferences than most other groups of workers for the hours supplied to be concentrated within specific time periods that are compatible with these commitments. Nurses also appear to exhibit a much stronger preference for some of the non-pecuniary aspects of the job than do other workers.

There are several important dimensions to the labour supply of nursing. First the decision to invest in the human capital required to enter the occupation; this dimension involves the theory of occupational choice. Second the decision, conditional on occupational choice, whether or not to work. This participation decision has prominent life-cycle elements, reflecting the optimal timing of withdrawals from work for child-bearing and child-rearing purposes. Finally, conditional on the participation, is the decision on hours of work. Consider each of these in turn.

OCCUPATIONAL CHOICE

The long-run determinants of the supply of nurses are modelled within the theory of occupational choice. Empirically the choice of occupation can be modelled as either a binary choice between nursing and all other occupations or as a multinomial choice between nursing and a range of other separately identified occupations. Lifetime utility is maximized subject to a lifetime budget constraint. Lifetime consumption and leisure enter as determinants of lifetime utility while expected net lifetime wage rates, expected lifetime years and hours of work enter the budget constraint. Expected net lifetime wage rates result from a comparison of the expected earnings in nursing and the other occupations considered and the scale of the required human capital investment in nursing and the other occupations considered. The choice of the occupation nursing, N, can then be explained by a set of variables which capture expected net lifetime wage rates, En/Y, where these have been appropriately discounted, individual characteristics, X, and perhaps household or parental characteristics, P, which influence choice. Thus:

$$N = f(En/Y, X, P) \tag{6.1}$$

PARTICIPATION AND HOURS OF WORK

The classic labour supply model is based on an individual's supply of hours of work, conditional on their participation in the workforce (Killingsworth 1983). Labour supply is seen as a function of a set of independent variables. The classic model assumes that the most important among these is the wage rate (W). Other important determinants are likely to be other, non-labour, income, V (income from other sources and the income of the spouse), non-pecuniary job characteristics (Z), and sociodemographic and individual worker characteristics (S), which may be unobservable, which account for differences in tastes. Thus:

$$H = f(W, V, Z, S) \tag{6.2}$$

This specification can be derived from a direct utility function, by solving the first-order conditions for a maximum and obtaining the demand for leisure (and therefore for hours of work). It is simplest to view consumption opportunities as summarized within a composite consumer good. Assume the following quasi-concave utility function:

$$U(C_t, L_t, X_t) \tag{6.3}$$

in which C_t, L_t and X_t are within-period consumption, leisure hours and individual attributes, respectively, in period t. Utility is maximized subject to the budget constraint:

$$C_t + W_t L_t = V_t + W_t T \tag{6.4}$$

where T is the total time available and hours of work, H, are therefore given by $H = T - L$. The Lagrangian function and first-order conditions take the form:

$$\psi = U(C_t, L_t, X_t) - \lambda[(C_t - V_t - W_t(T - L_t))] \tag{6.5}$$

$$U_C(C_t, L_t, X_t) = \lambda \quad U_L(C_t, L_t, X_t) \geqslant \lambda W_t \quad \text{or} \quad \frac{U_L}{U_C} \geqslant W_t \tag{6.6}$$

If the equality holds, we have an interior solution where $L_t < T$ and the individual participates in the labour force. On the other hand if the inequality holds strictly, then the individual is not working (corner solution). The wage (W_r) is the reservation wage, such that $U_L(C_t, L_t, X_t) = \lambda W_r$, below which the individual will not work. The reservation wage is equal to the marginal rate of substitution evaluated at $H = 0$.

The marginal rate of substitution between goods and leisure (M) is:

$$M \equiv \frac{(\partial U/\partial L)}{(\partial U/\partial C)} = M(WH + V, 1 - H, e) \qquad (6.7)$$

The individual will work if $W - W_r = 0$. Optimal hours of work are where W equals M.

Labour supply decisions are taken in a family or household context and will be affected by income tax and welfare benefits. The standard 'unitary' family labour supply model treats the family of two working-age individuals as a single decision-making unit. The utility function may then be written:

$$U_t(C_t, L_{1t}, L_{2t}, X_t) \qquad (6.8)$$

where L_{1t} and L_{2t} are the leisure of the two family members and children and other dependants are included in the vector of household attributes, X_t. Full income is now given by:

$$M_t = V_t + W_{1t}T + W_{2t}\, T \qquad (6.9)$$

and reservation wages can be computed for each family as above. Demand for leisure, and therefore hours of work, now take the form:

$$L_{1t} = L_1(W_{1t}, W_{2t}, M_t, X_t) \leqslant T \qquad L_{2t} = L_2(W_{1t}, W_{2t}, M_t, X_t) \leqslant T \qquad (6.10)$$

The 'unitary' approach to household labour supply entails some restrictions which are often considered to be unreasonable (Slutsky symmetry and income pooling). A popular alternative framework is the 'collective' model that relaxes the income allocation rule among individuals so that this allocation will reflect the bargaining positions of individuals within the family.

PROBLEMS IN ESTIMATION OF LABOUR SUPPLY

Empirical work in the general area of labour supply has encountered three main problems which are of concern when seeking to estimate the labour supply of nurses. Each of these are discussed below.

SAMPLE SELECTION

When estimating short-run labour supply functions for nurses a potential bias arises in the estimates of the nursing labour supply elasticities because of the exclusion of non-working nurses from the sample. The researcher cannot observe the potential hours of work of non-working nurses and thus the data on hours are censored. The employees captured in the sample have lower reservation wages, place a greater value on work, and therefore offer more hours of work at the prevailing wage rates than the population as a whole. Evidently the population captured in the sample differs from the population as a whole with respect to unobservable individual characteristics, tastes or preferences for work. Thus the data on recorded hours worked are censored and the error term for the recorded subsample of workers may not be a mean-zero random variable. Instead it tends to be positive even though it is a mean-zero random variable in the population as a whole. Applying ordinary least squares (OLS) to a sample limited to those who work implies that coefficients will be biased downward and inconsistent; the resulting reservation wage will be lower and the regression line will be flatter than the true one.

Sample selection issues can be addressed using the well-known Heckman procedure. The conditional expectation of hours worked for those employed can be written as:

$$E(H|H \succ 0) = X_i\beta + \sigma\lambda_i \qquad (6.11)$$

where X_i is a vector of independent variables, including the wage and other socio-economic characteristics, and the σ in the second term, the error term for the recorded subsample, is non-zero. Exclusion of the latter term can be viewed as an omitted variable problem in a linear hours-worked regression equation. Heckman (1979) suggests adding λ_i, the inverse Mill's ratio, as a regressor to the hours equation before carrying out OLS estimation on the working sample of an individual, where λ is generated by a subsidiary equation which estimates labour market participation as follows. Suppose there is an underlying response variable, P^*, which represents true labour market participation:

$$P^* = aX_i + u_i \qquad (6.12)$$

where X_i is a vector of variables determining coverage and a is a vector of parameters. P^* is not observable but $P = 1$ if $P^* = aX_i + u_i > 0$ and otherwise $P = 0$. This observed binary variable P now forms the basis for a reduced form probit equation of the participation decision allowing the construction of the inverse Mill's ratio, λ_i, where:

$$\lambda = -\frac{\phi}{\Phi} \quad \text{for participation}$$

where ϕ = standard normal density function and Φ = cumulative distribution function. λ is then included in the OLS estimate of the determinants of hours of work. Inclusion of Mill's ratio makes estimation consistent.

MEASUREMENT ERROR

Measurement error results from the type of data available on pay. There are a number of different dimensions to this problem. First where pay is self-reported it can be reported with error for respondents may not keep detailed records of what they are paid. In general, employer reporting of pay provides more accurate data because employers keep detailed records (Mellow & Sider 1983). However these same records often fail to record all the hours employees work because employers only record the hours they pay for. Typically they do not offer overtime pay to non-manual employees and therefore they do not record any hours they work in excess of the standard working week. Thus where the current hourly wage is computed by taking the ratio of annual or weekly pay to annual or weekly hours of work, and the computation uses employer reported data, there may be measurement error because hours of work are under-recorded. One consequence of this type of measurement error is that it will overstate the hourly rates of pay of non-manual employees who are of course the employees on the highest rates of pay. This method of calculating the hourly rate of pay also means that any errors in the measurement of labour supply will be duplicated in the constructed measure of pay and this will give rise to a spurious correlation. The technique of instrumental variables has often been used to overcome this errors-in-variables problem.

The hourly wage required for estimation is the net of tax marginal wage. In the presence of progressive taxation this diverges from the average wage, but the most commonly available measures of pay allow for only the computation of the average wage. Where the individual works beyond a particular number of hours under a progressive tax system the average after-tax hourly wage will be greater than the after-tax marginal wage. Estimating an hours of work equation using the average rate of pay will therefore introduce a potential negative bias on the relative coefficient.

THE FUNCTIONAL FORM OF THE ESTIMATED MODEL

Although generated from the same individual preference functions, the appropriate specification of the hours of work equation and the participation equation are very different. It is not possible to use the same model to analyse the two different dimensions of labour supply. We saw above that in order to estimate hours worked a regression method which deals with censored distributions is required, that is, a sample selection-corrected regression is required. For participation, binomial or multinomial logit and probit models are preferred because they are efficient and robust against non-normality and heteroscedasticity. They constrain the dependent variable to integer values.

EVOLUTION OF EMPIRICAL RESEARCH INTO LABOUR SUPPLY

Empirical work into the labour supply of nurses has evolved in line with more general models of labour supply. Early empirical work into the labour supply of nurses utilized *ad hoc* models and simple estimation methods, such as OLS or 2SLS, 3SLS. The functional forms were not derived explicitly from utility or indirect utility functions. The models did not address issues such as corner solutions[1] and problems related to the error term (sample selection bias). Estimates of intra-family or cross-substitution elasticities, the income-compensated effects of a unit change in the wage of the spouse on the labour supply of the nurse, were very rare in these studies. The common simplifying assumption was that cross-substitution effects were zero. The elasticities produced by these studies ranged from 0.54 to 0.89 for the USA (see Brewer 1998) but are not reliable because of the above problems of model estimation. This said, there appears to be less variation in the elasticities which were estimated for nurses than in those estimated for female labour supply as a whole; estimates of the latter range from -0.10 to $+1.60$ (see Ashenfelter & Card 1999).

Considerable progress was subsequently made on both the functional form of the labour supply model and the estimation techniques. Supply equations, derived explicitly from a utility function, were more complete, thus reducing the biases produced by omitted variables. Twin linear probability models (Sloan & Richupan 1975) and Tobit models (Sloan & Richupan 1975; Link & Settle 1980, 1985) were employed. The twin linear probability models first estimated participation using a linear probability model and the complete sample of working and non-working individuals recorded in the data set. They then used the subsample of participants, to estimate the amount of time worked using a linear regression model. Like OLS these models did not deal with censored distributions but this shortcoming was overcome by the use of Tobit models. These models also began to address issues of sample selection using Heckman's procedure.

While evolving in terms of estimation technique, empirical work now also began to investigate a range of additional issues. The own wage responsiveness by age and race cohort was estimated by Link and Settle (1980). Others included variables measuring nurses' subjective evaluations of their working environment, such as lack of participation in decisions, provision of day care facilities and occupational ladders, as well as relative wages, in the hours of work equation (see Bahrami 1988).

[1] Corner solutions to maximization problems in a labour supply model arise when the desired hours of work are negative, or in other words, where the reservation wage is higher than the market wage. In this case, a complete model of labour supply should set the actual hours worked equal to zero, and a corner solution arises.

At this time more general models of women's labour supply addressed a range of wider issues of considerable relevance to empirical work on nurses. When examining the labour supply behaviour of married women these studies highlighted the fixed costs of labour market entry, the costs of transportation and childcare arrangements and the expenses necessarily incurred in the performance of the job. Such fixed costs introduce discontinuities into the labour supply function, because women will only start working beyond some positive minimum number of hours, the reservation hours, which generate an income from work sufficient to cover these fixed costs (see Blank 1988; Cogan 1980). More recently, Blundell *et al.* (1998) have emphasized the importance of distinguishing between the impact of fixed costs and search costs on the participation decision. They show that business cycle variables affect the participation decision through their impact on search costs. Models which ignore the potential discontinuity in supply, which results from the presence of fixed costs, may overestimate substantially the parameters that underlie married women's labour supply behaviour. In spite of the importance of this issue, only two studies have, to the knowledge of these authors, allowed for discontinuities when focusing on nurses' labour supply (see Phillips 1995; Skåtun *et al.* 2001).

EMPIRICAL EVIDENCE FROM THE LATE 1980s AND 1990s

THE USA

Many of the recent studies of nursing labour supply in the USA have utilized data from the quadrennial National Sample Survey of Registered Nurses (NSSRN). These studies have addressed issues such as part-time vs. full-time labour supply and the labour supply of male nurses using advanced econometric techniques.

Brewer (1996) used the 1984 and 1988 NSSRN to examine the labour supply response of Registered Nurses in the USA at different stages of the economic cycle. The determinants of annual hours were estimated using OLS, while participation was estimated using a logistic regression in which the choices modelled were between not working, part-time working and full-time working. Wages were instrumented for working and non-working nurses to prevent bias in the OLS regression. The results revealed that female nurses were more responsive to changes in own wage under the shortage conditions that prevailed in 1988, when the elasticity was 1.45, than they were in 1984 under what was termed market equilibrium, when the elasticity was 1.35.

Mallikamas (1990) used the 1984 and 1988 NSSRN to estimate a nested logit model where the choices were between either working as a nurse full time or part time, and then conditional on working as a nurse, either working in a hospital or not in a hospital. The choices of hours of work and specialty, if working in a hospital, were also modelled. Own wage rate and the degree of autonomy afforded by nursing jobs were found to be important factors determining participation, although these were insignificant determinants of the choice of part-time working, choice of hours of work and choice of specialty. Own wage elasticity was again found to be higher in 1988, at 1.21, than in 1984, when it was 0.90.

Link (1992) analysed the determinants of the labour force participation and hours of work of Registered Nurses over the period 1960–1988 using Heckman's procedure to correct for sample selection. The presence of selection bias was tested for but found not to be significant in all years other than 1977. The own wage elasticities of married working nurses were found to be insignificant for all years except 1988, and the values ranged from −0.39 to 0.19, much lower than the estimates reported above. This study also reported that the participation rate for nurses was greater than 87%, which was higher than that for females in general as well as that of prime-age males.

Laing and Rademaker (1990) used stepwise regression to estimate hours of work and stepwise discriminant analyses to distinguish between three categories of workforce attachment: full-time working, part-time working and without work. The analysis sought to rank the factors influencing married nurses' labour force participation. A measure of the division of labour within the family, labelled 'sex role attitude', was found to be the strongest predictor of participation. Among the economic variables, only the spouse's salary was an important predictor of participation, while a nurse's own wage was not significant in any of the models.

Lehrer *et al.* (1991) found that the provision of employer-sponsored child-care had a positive and significant impact on hours worked per year by Registered Nurses with young children. Using 1988 data the authors found evidence of an increase in reported attachment to the employer as a result of the availability of childcare facilities which they estimated was roughly equivalent to that associated with a wage raise of $6 per hour.

Ault and Rutman (1994) emphasize the sensitivity of results derived to different measures of labour supply. Labour supply can be defined in terms of either annual hours of work or weeks worked per year. Using a probit and 2SLS model, and correcting for sample heterogeneity, they find that own wage rates are insignificant determinants of labour supply. Moreover the presence of other income and of children are more significant determinants of the choice between full-time and part-time working than they are of the decision to work or not to work.

To summarize, empirical studies conducted in the 1990s reveal considerable diversity over the sign, size and significance of the variables determining nursing labour supply in the USA. Estimates are sensitive to the econometric and statistical assumptions made and hence to model specification. More recent studies seem to have cast doubt over the role of own wages in labour supply.

THE UK

Very little empirical research has been conducted into nursing labour supply in the UK. The authors are aware of only two studies which investigate this issue using advanced econometric techniques based on the classic model of labour supply; these studies are Phillips (1995) and Skåtun *et al.* (2001).

The first of these, Phillips (1995), investigated the presence of discontinuities in the labour supply curve arising from the fixed costs associated with work, where these costs are understood to be greatest for married women. The base model was neoclassical, the decision to work depended upon a comparison between the reservation wage and the market wage. A selection bias-corrected probit model was used to estimate the probability of labour market participation by a nurse and a selection bias-corrected OLS regression was used to estimate their hours of work. The data on British nurses were drawn from the Women and Employment Survey in 1980, but the resulting sample size was small, 312, after rejecting observations subject to miscoding errors and/or missing values.

The study revealed an elasticity of participation with respect to the wage of 1.4 and an elasticity of participation with respect to non-labour income of −0.38. The own wage elasticity of hours of work was small at 0.15. The study tested for discontinuities in the supply function resulting from the presence of fixed costs. Reservation hours were estimated to be 15.8 per week, while the elasticity of participation with respect to changes in these fixed costs of working was estimated to be −0.67 for all the nurses, although slightly lower at −0.64 for married nurses. The author concludes that changes in wages are likely to be an effective way of managing the supply of nurses, at least where participation rates are not high and as a result 'allow room for response' (Phillips 1985). The author also concludes that policies to reduce working costs, perhaps the provision of creche or other childcare facilities, may also produce small gains in participation.

The second study by Skåtun *et al.* (2001) estimated participation and hours of work by married or co-habiting qualified nurses in the UK using the Quarterly Labour Force Survey for 1999–2000. The sample comprises 1248 people who held a nursing qualification at that time. The study used a two-step selection bias-corrected Heckman wage equation to estimate hours of work. Estimates of the inverse Mill's ratio were obtained from a probit participation equation and included in the OLS estimation of hours of work. A second and main participation equation was estimated using a logit model. The study found that the own wage elasticity of participation was positive and inelastic at 0.62 and that participation was also inelastic, and as predicted negative, with respect to partner's wage and non-labour income, where these were −0.12 and −0.009 respectively. The own wage elasticity of hours of work was found to be inelastic at 0.48. The authors conclude that both changes in wages and childcare policies affect the labour supply of married nurses.

It is noteworthy that the elasticities derived in this second study differ from those estimated by Phillips (1995) and reported above. The own wage elasticity of participation is smaller than that in Phillips, while the own wage elasticity of hours of work is larger, at almost three times the size, than that estimated by Phillips. In the second study the elasticities of both participation and hours of work are inelastic, < 1. However they are still sufficiently large to suggest that pay plays an important role in decisions on participation and hours of work. A 1% rise in the real, relative, pay of nurses for a workforce of 450,000 working an average 40 hours per week would encourage almost 3000 more to work and produce in total over 86,000 additional hours ($0.48\% \times 40 \times 450,000$).

The remaining studies for the UK have focused on different aspects of labour supply. In a series of papers Gray et al. (1996) and Gray and Phillips (1994, 1996) have analysed nursing labour turnover. Gray and Phillips (1996) found that two local labour market variables were significantly related to turnover across all staff groups. These were the size of the private health care sector and the relative pay with respect to the local average for comparable workers. Gray et al. (1996) investigated the impact of pay on turnover and concluded that across the board, national pay increases were not generally a cost-effective way of reducing turnover rates. Gray and Phillips (1994) studied the relationship between age, length of service and turnover rates among different NHS staff groups, among which were nurses. They found that, in common with other occupations, turnover rates declined with age and were highest in the first years of service.

A series of surveys commissioned by the Royal College of Nursing (RCN) and conducted by Seccombe and Smith (1996, 1997) have contributed to our understanding of the characteristics of the nursing labour market and the motivation of individual nursing, but none has taken what could be termed a 'rounded' assessment of supply and demand issues.

STUDIES OF JOB SATISFACTION AND NURSING LABOUR SUPPLY

An indirect way of estimating the labour supply is through analysis of job satisfaction. Theoretical models link an individual's labour supply to pecuniary and non-pecuniary job characteristics. However, the role of the non-pecuniary job characteristics, such as promotion and training opportunities, the flexibility of working hours, job security and control over hours of work, which the theory of compensating differentials would suggest should be included, have been largely neglected in the traditional empirical literature, which has focused on the role of wages. The impact of pecuniary and non-pecuniary job characteristics on labour supply has been investigated through the econometric analysis of job satisfaction. This research has also attempted to examine the relationship between job satisfaction and indirect measures of labour supply such as turnover, absenteeism and decisions to quit.

The economic literature examining the relationship between job satisfaction and quitting behaviour is scant. The explanation for this is the lack of large longitudinal data sets which enable the researcher to identify job satisfaction at time $t-1$ and job turnover at some subsequent time t. The first general study by Freeman (1978) used panel data from the US National Longitudinal Survey and the Michigan Panel Survey of Income Dynamics. The author found that job satisfaction was a significant determinant of quitting and was quantitatively more important than wages.

Shields and Ward (2001) conducted the only analysis of nursing job satisfaction and labour turnover for the UK. The study drew on a large and unique national survey of NHS nursing staff collected in 1994; the sample size was 9625. The researchers ran an ordered probit model to explain job satisfaction. Those more likely to be found dissatisfied were the young, males, those from ethnic minorities and the more highly educated among NHS nurses. Those nurses emphasizing the more pecuniary aspects of the job reported lower levels of job satisfaction and relatively low pay was found to be a source of dissatisfaction.

The authors also estimated a binary probit model in order to identify the determinants of the declared intention to leave the NHS in the three years following interview. Nurses who reported overall dissatisfaction with their jobs had a 65% higher probability of intending to quit than those reporting to be satisfied. Principal component analysis showed that low morale linked to poor career advancement and training opportunities had a greater impact on intentions to quit than either workload or pay. A more recent study by one of the authors (Shields & Price 2002) reveals that perceptions of racial harassment by nurses from ethnic minorities is one source of dissatisfaction resulting in intentions to quit.

THE DEMAND FOR NURSING SERVICES

The wages we observe for nurses are the result of factors on both the supply and the demand side of the labour market. Thus we turn now to look at the labour demand side of the market. The demand for nursing services in the UK is dominated by the NHS, and the amount of labour it buys is determined by the size of NHS budgets, the price of nursing services and the availability and price of other complementary and substitute factors of production. The demand for nursing services, in common with the demand for all other types of labour, is a derived demand; it is derived from the final demand for the output that the labour produces. Though this demand for health care services originates with the UK public it is moderated, in the case of a publicly provided health service like that in the UK, by the expenditures that the government is willing to devote to these services. It is easy to understand that, other things equal, the demand for nursing services will be greater the greater the level of expenditure the government is willing to commit to health care services, and that all other things equal it will be greater the lower the price of nursing, the lower are nurses' wages or any of the other non-pecuniary elements (pensions, etc.) that add to nurses' labour costs. The demand for nursing will also be greater, again all other things equal, the less easy it is to substitute the services that nurses provide by either technology or the services of other health care professionals, and the easier it is to substitute the services that other health service professionals provide at higher prices by services provided by nurses. Finally it is also clear that, all other things equal, the demand for nursing services will be greater the more readily available is the supply of those other complementary inputs to nursing services, such as for example hospital beds for those nursing services delivered in hospitals.

The demand for nurses' services can be modelled as a downward-sloping labour demand curve. The position of that curve is determined by the levels of expenditure the government commits to health services, while the slope is determined by the responsiveness of the quantity demanded to any change in the price of nursing services – by the elasticity of demand for nursing services. Some of the factors listed above, the availability of complements and substitutes, will be determinants of this elasticity. More generally the determinants of the elasticity of demand for all types of labour have been summarized in the Hicks–Marshall rules of derived demand. These state that, all other things equal, the own wage elasticity of demand for labour will be smaller, i.e. will be less elastic:

(i) The smaller is the absolute value of the price elasticity of demand for the final product the labour produces;
(ii) The more difficult it is to substitute other factors of production for labour;
(iii) The less elastic is the supply of other substitute factors of production;
(iv) The smaller is the share of labour in total costs. Though subsequently Hicks showed that this condition may not always hold.

Considering each of these in turn, in the specific context of the market for nursing services, enables us to understand the ultimate determinants of the demand for the labour services of nurses.

The first rule may be interpreted as stating that if it is difficult for consumers to substitute other types of services for health services, then the value of the price elasticity of demand for health services, and therefore the own wage elasticity of the derived demand for nursing services, will be small. The elasticity will be small if when nurses' wages rise and as a result push up the price of health services, consumers have little choice but to pay the higher price and continue consuming the services provided by nurses. This would be the case if there were no adequate substitutes for nursing services. However most of the health services that are produced by nurses are not priced, they are free to the consumer at the point of consumption. How does this affect the argument?

In the private health sector nurses' pay directly affects the price of health services charged to the consumer even though consumers may be shielded from the short-run consequences of a pay rise if the health plan absorbs the rise in the price of health services. In the long run however the pay rise will be passed on to the consumer in the form of higher health plan costs. So there is long-run elasticity to consider. In the public sector health services are provided free at point of consumption and paid for out of taxation. In the public sector the consequences of a rise in nurses' pay could therefore be either higher taxes or lower output of other public services if the government decides not to increase taxation. In the short run the consumer may be shielded from these consequences for they may have little immediate impact on the volume or quality of public services, but they will emerge in the long run. However in the short run any rise in nurses' pay will have important consequences for the consumers' agent, the government. They will have to decide whether to fund the pay rise and if they do, whether to pay for this by either reducing expenditure on other items or by increasing taxation. How much employment falls as a result of any pay rise depends on how much of the pay rise the government decides to fund. This determinant of the elasticity of derived demand for nursing services therefore depends on the government's willingness to fund pay rises for nurses. During the 1990s governments proved reluctant to fund large pay rises for nurses.

The second rule explores both the possibilities of allowing other health care workers and even technology to provide the services presently supplied by nurses and of allowing nurses to supply some of the services presently provided by doctors. It encompasses both the possibility of substituting domestically trained nurses by foreign trained nurses and of some senior nurses undertaking some of the tasks undertaken by GPs and hospital doctors (see Chapter 10). The opportunities for the former would seem to be high, as evidenced by the importation of large numbers of foreign trained nurses into the NHS in England. The latter is only now beginning to be explored by some health boards and is encountering resistance from the professional organizations representing doctors. A number of health boards in England are also now employing care assistants to perform some of the more routine tasks previously performed by trained nurses, and the Wanless Report advocates further scrutiny of the opportunities for such substitution. If trained nurses wish to protect or improve their wages it is in their interests to seek to reduce these substitution possibilities, to argue for total patient care and resist the stripping out of more routine parts of their jobs. Similar arguments are also likely to be advanced by doctors as they seek to protect their pay by minimizing the opportunities for nurses undertaking some of their duties. The substitution possibilities at both these margins are however likely to be increasingly closely scrutinized and exploited over the next few years.

The third rule emphasizes that even where the substitution possibilities discussed above exist these may be difficult to achieve if, when attempted, the price of these substitutes rises sharply because they are in inelastic supply. Any sharp rise in the price of the substitute labour would make it less attractive and deter the substitution. But suppose there were a ready supply of people willing to work as care assistants or of foreign trained nurses willing to work in the UK, at the prevailing rates of pay, then there would be no barrier on grounds of cost to realizing these substitution possibilities. The supply of these substitute workers would be highly elastic and there would be no price barriers to substitution. At the time of writing this seems to be the case with foreign trained nurses, though it is less clear how large is the pool of people willing to work as care assistants.

The fourth and final rule as originally stated by Marshall has been termed the 'importance of being unimportant'. If the labour in question accounts for only a small part of total costs even a very substantial rise in wage costs will have little effect on overall cost and therefore on the final price of the product. However this is evidently not the case with nurses for they account for a very substantial proportion of the total NHS pay bill and any rise in nurses' pay will have a substantial impact on the total NHS pay bill and therefore on total NHS costs.

Thus it can be concluded that the own wage elasticity of demand for nurses, in particular for domestically trained nurses, is likely to be quite high in the medium to long run. In the medium to long run there appears to be an elastic supply of substitute foreign trained nurses, while there are also ready substitutes, in the form of care assistants, for some of the tasks presently performed by nurses. Whether these substitution possibilities will be realized will depend on the decisions of health service managers and the political will of governments. If these substitution possibilities were realized they would be expected to put downward pressure on nurses' pay, without any deterioration in either the quality or quantity of nursing services supplied. However the demand for some other types of nursing services may prove less elastic where they offer a cheap alternative to some of the services currently provided by doctors. This may provide a countervailing source of upward pressure on pay for some nurses.

What do we know about the values of the key parameters of the nurses' labour demand function? The answer is nothing, for there have been no empirical estimates of the values of either the own wage elasticity of labour demand or the elasticity of demand for nurses with respect to the price of other inputs for the UK. It is perhaps not surprising, in view of the institutional complexities, that this has proved such an unattractive research area, but it is to be hoped that some work will shortly be undertaken to better inform public policy on this matter.

NURSES' PAY

In the UK the demand for nursing services originates from the NHS and the private health service sector. However the NHS is the dominant player and in many parts of the country is the single source of demand for nursing services. Though the NHS comprises many different trusts and health boards, when setting pay they act as a single body. This monopsony power of the NHS is confronted on the supply side by the trade union representing nurses, the Royal College of Nursing (RCN). The RCN represents nurses in wage bargaining and assumes many of the characteristics of a monopoly seller of labour.

The institutional arrangements for setting pay have reinforced the monopoly power of the RCN. Since 1984 national, UK wide, rates of pay have been established as a result of the deliberations of the Review Body for Nursing Staff, Midwives, Health Visitors and Professions Allied to Medicine. These institutional arrangements have been constructed to mediate the power of the two sides in pay setting and to reduce the opportunities for the exploitations of either monopoly or monopsony power. These national rates of pay have exhibited very little regional variation. However this may change, perhaps as a result of increasing divergence in conditions in local and regional labour markets, for where this happens it will reduce the enthusiasm of the NHS employers for national rates of pay.

There are very few systematic studies of nurses' pay. Elliott and Duffus (1996) reported trends in the relative pay of nurses over the period 1970 to 1992. Using data on pay settlements and New Earnings Survey data on earnings, they mapped the trends in real pay and the size of wage settlement over this period. They also reported the scale of wage drift: the difference between the increase in earnings and the size of the pay settlements awarded in any period. They showed that nurses enjoyed one of the fastest rates of growth of earnings of any group of public sector workers over the period. Yet despite this they also showed that the earnings of female nurses deteriorated over the period 1980 to 1993 relative to non-manual workers in the economy as a whole. Though the analysis of Elliott and Duffus enables us to distinguish trends in relative pay it does not enable us to distinguish the causes of the underlying pay differentials, because it does not control for differences in the productive characteristics of nurses and the groups with whom they are being compared.

Nor does it control for the differences in the characteristics of jobs done by nurses and their comparators.

Similar criticisms could be levelled against the recent exercise by Nickell and Quintini (2002) who once again use New Earnings Survey data. They report changes in the relative ranking of different groups of public sector workers in the overall earnings distribution. They show that despite the pay rises female nurses have achieved over the period 1975 to 1999, these were not sufficient to maintain their position in the overall female earnings distribution. In the period 1975–79 the earnings of female nurses aged between 31 and 40 were sufficient to place them in the 64th percentile in the overall distribution of earnings for all female workers aged 31 to 40. By the period 1985–89 they had slipped to the 57th percentile and by 1999 to the 56th. The decline in pay relative to that of other females of the same age appears to have occurred during the late 1970s and the first half of the 1980s and the position has altered little since then.

These authors then proceed to assess whether this decline in relative pay has meant a decline in workforce quality. Using the results of test scores from the National Child Development Survey (NCDS) they test whether there has also been a decline in the average percentile position, in the ranking by attainment in these tests, between those entering nursing in the late 1970s and those entering in the early 1990s. They find a small but statistically insignificant decline in ranking over this period. There is therefore no empirical support for the proposition that the decline in relative pay has been associated with a decline in the quality of entrants to nursing.

A recent study by Morris and McGuire (2001) attempts to control for differences in the productive characteristics of nurses and their comparators. Using data from the Quarterly Labour Force Survey from Spring 1997 to Autumn 2000 they identify 4511 individuals who hold a nursing qualification (coded into Standard Occupational Classification code 340). They then estimate a double selectivity model, to allow for both occupational choice, and among those who have chosen to acquire the human capital necessary to become a nurse, the participation decision.

Evidently a standard OLS estimate of the pay differential between nurses and other workers might suffer from bias if those who have chosen nursing as a career, and those from amongst this number who have chosen to work, do not constitute a random draw from the underlying population. Those who have chosen nursing as a career may have a greater aptitude or ability for nursing than the population in general, thus they will be more productive in nursing jobs than would a random sample from the population. Again those who choose to work as nurses may have different reservation wages and productivity than the population in general. For these reasons a simple OLS comparison of nurses' pay with that of other workers may produce a biased estimate of the pay premium in nursing.

The results of the study should best be regarded as provisional for the controls included by the authors may not adequately capture differences in human capital, and characteristics of the jobs done by nurses and other workers. It is nonetheless interesting to note that they find that nurses receive on average 33% higher hourly wages than other, comparable workers. Not surprisingly therefore these same authors (Morris & McGuire 2002) discover a high private rate of return to the investment required to become a nurse.

CONCLUSIONS

Evidently substantially more work remains to be done in the areas of labour demand and relative pay. We know little of either the true magnitude of any pay differential enjoyed by nurses or how this has changed over the years. We know even less about several important aspects of the labour demand for nurses, i.e. the own wage elasticity of labour demand or the elasticity of demand with respect to other factor prices. There has been very little research into the degree of, or opportunities for, substitution between care assistants and nurses on the one hand and between nurses and doctors on the other. How substantial has such substitution been and have changing pay relativities or technological change been the drivers of such substitution?

We know a bit more about labour supply but UK empirical research on nursing labour supply has still been scarce. There is a need for research into the major drivers of behaviour in the nursing labour market. Biased parameter estimates can result from omitted variables. The role of non-pecuniary job characteristics, and their importance relative to pecuniary job characteristics, need to be integrated within the more traditional labour supply models, for we know little of the relative importance of pay and these other factors. For the future advanced models of labour supply need to be constructed.[2] Research needs to extend beyond the standard static within-period labour supply framework, to multiperiod models in which labour supply is part of a lifetime decision-making process.

There is also a specific Scottish angle to this research. Scotland employs many more nurses per head of the population than England, so what do these extra nurses do? Is the occupational structure of the health service in Scotland different to that in England or does Scotland simply employ more of all types of health care professionals, in the same proportions as in England, because of its greater health needs? If however the production function for health care services, the proportions in which inputs are combined to produce health care services, is different in Scotland from that in England, is this a production function that England will come to adopt as it increases the share of its GDP that it spends on health care to the level in Scotland?

---

[2] For a comprehensive review of the most recent alternative approaches to labour supply see Ashenfelter and Card (1999), volume 3A, chapter 27.

ACKNOWLEDGEMENTS

The authors are particularly grateful to Alastair Gray for his perceptive and constructive comments on an earlier version of this chapter, to Tony Scott for permission to cite research conducted by him with the three authors of this chapter (see Antonazzo et al. 2002), to participants at a workshop held to discuss the contributions to this book to Alastair McGuire, Stephen Morris and to Alan Maynard for helpful comments. The Health Economics Research Unit is funded by the Chief Scientist Office of the Scottish Executive Health Department. The views are those of the authors and not the funders.

REFERENCES

Antonazzo E, Scott A, Skåtun D and Elliott RF (2002) The labour market for nursing: a review of the labour supply literature. *Health Economics* (forthcoming).

Ashenfelter O and Card D (1999) *Handbook of Labor Economics, Volume 3*. North-Holland, Amsterdam.

Ault DE and Rutman GL (1994) On selecting a measure of labour activity: evidence from registered nurses, 1981 and 1989. *Applied Economics*, **26**, 851–863.

Bahrami B (1988) Hours of work offered by nurses. *The Social Science Journal*, **25**(3), 325–335.

Blank RM (1988) Simultaneously modelling the supply of weeks and hours of work among female household heads. *Journal of Labor Economics*, **6**(2), 177–204.

Blundell R, Ham J and Meghir C (1998) Unemployment, discouraged workers and female labour supply. *Research in Economics*, **52**, 103–131.

Brewer CS (1996) The roller coaster supply of registered nurses: lessons from the eighties. *Research in Nursing & Health*, **19**, 345–357.

Brewer CS (1998) The history and future of nursing labour research in a cost control environment. *Research in Nursing and Health*, **21**, 167–177.

Cogan J (1980) Labor supply with costs of labor market entry. In GP Smith (Ed.), *Female Labor Supply: Theory and Estimation*. Princeton University Press, Princeton, NJ, pp. 327–359.

Elliott RF and Duffus K (1996) What has been happening to pay in this public sector of the British economy? Developments over the period 1990–1992. *British Journal of Industrial Relations*, **34**(1), 51–86.

Elliott RF, Mavromaras K, Scott A, Bell DNF, Antonazzo E, Gerova V and van der Pol M (2002) *Labour markets and NHS Scotland*. Report to the Scottish Executive Central Research Unit, University of Aberdeen, Aberdeen.

Freeman RB (1978) Job satisfaction as an economic variable. *American Economic Review*, **68**, 135–141.

Gray A and Phillips VL (1994) Turnover, age and length of service: a comparison of nurses and other staff in the National Health Service. *Journal of Advanced Nursing*, **19**, 819–827.

Gray A and Phillips VL (1996) Labour turnover in the British National Health Service: a labour market analysis. *Health Policy*, **36**, 273–289.

Gray A, Phillips VL and Normand C (1996) The cost of turnover: evidence from the British National Health Service. *Health Policy*, **38**, 117–128.

Health Departments for Great Britain (2001) Written evidence for the Review Body for Nursing Staff, Midwives, Health Visitors and Professions Allied to Medicine – Review for 2002. Health Departments of Great Britain, London.

Heckman JJ (1979) Sample selection bias as a specification error. *Econometrica*, **47**, 153–162.

Killingsworth MR (1983) *Labour Supply*. Cambridge University Press, Cambridge.

Laing GP and Rademaker AW (1990) Married registered nurses' labour force participation. *The Canadian Journal of Nursing Research*, **22**(1), 21–38.

Lehrer E, Santero T and Mohan-Neill S (1991) The impact of employer-sponsored child care on female labour supply behaviour: evidence from the nursing profession. *Population Research and Policy Review*, **10**, 197–212.

Link CR (1992) Labor supply behavior of registered nurses: female labor supply in the future? *Research in Labor Economics*, **13**, 287–320.

Link CR and Settle RF (1980) Financial incentive and labor supply of married professional nurses: an economic analysis. *Nursing Research*, **29**(4), 238–243.

Link CR and Settle RF (1985) Labor supply responses of licensed practical nurses: a partial solution to a nurse shortage? *Journal of Economics and Business*, **37**, 49–57.

Mallikamas S (1990) *Short run labor supply of registered nurses*. PhD Thesis, University of Wisconsin.

Mellow W and Sider H (1983) Accuracy of responses in labor market surveys: evidence and implications. *Journal of Labor Economics*, **1**, 33–44.

Morris S and McGuire A (2001) *A double selectivity model of earnings for nurses in Great Britain*. Paper presented to Health Economists Study Group, City University.

Morris S and McGuire A (2002) *The net present value to becoming a nurse in Britain*. Mimeo, Department of Economics, City University, 34 pp.

Nickell S and Quintini G (2002) The consequences of the decline in public sector pay in Britain: a little bit of evidence. *Economic Journal*, **112**(477), 107–118.

Office of Health Economics (1999) *Compendium of Health Statistics*, 11th Edition.

Phillips VL (1995) Nurses labour supply: participation, hours of work, and discontinuities in the supply function. *Journal of Health Economics*, **14**, 567–582.

Rosen S (1986) The theory of equalising differences. In O Ashenfelter and PRG Layard (Eds), *Handbook of Labor Economics, Volume 11*. North-Holland, Amsterdam, pp. 641–692.

Seccombe I and Smith G (1996) *In the Balance: Registered Nurse Supply and Demand*. The Institute for Employment Studies, Report No. 315.

Seccombe I and Smith G (1997) *Taking part: registered nurses and the labour market in 1997*. The Institute for Employment Studies, Report No. 338.

Shields M and Ward M (2001) Improving nurse retention in the British National Health Service: the impact of job satisfaction on intentions to quit. *Journal of Health Economics*, **20**, 677–701.

Shields MA and Wheatley Price S (2002) Racial harassment, job satisfaction and intentions to quit: evidence from the British nursing profession. *Economica*, **69**, 295–326.

Skåtun D, Antonazzo E, Scott A and Elliott RF (2001) *Attracting qualified nurses back into nursing: an econometric analysis of nurses labour supply*. Paper presented at Department of Economics, University of Bergen.

Sloan FA and Richupan S (1975) Short-run supply responses of professional nurses: a microanalysis. *The Journal of Human Resources*, **10**, 242–257.

Smith A (1776) *The Wealth of Nations*, book 1, chapter X.

Wanless D (2002) *Securing our future health: taking a long-term view*. Final Report, April, Public Enquiry Unit, HM Treasury, London.

7

The Economics of the Hospital: Issues of Asymmetry and Uncertainty as they Affect Hospital Reimbursement

ALASTAIR McGUIRE
LSE Health and Social Care, LSE and King's College, London University

DAVID HUGHES
Department of Health

INTRODUCTION

Consideration of how hospitals ought to be reimbursed is not straightforward. Consider reimbursing the hospital for all the patients treated. The incentive for the hospital is to treat as many patients as possible. Hospitals might treat some patients who could be treated at lower cost elsewhere (for example, surgery to remove wisdom teeth or moles could be undertaken by dentists or GPs, saving resources for the health sector generally and possibly improving patient welfare by making access easier). Or it may lead to hospitals providing a quality of care that is higher than necessary. It is important, therefore, to set out the issues surrounding reimbursement clearly before considering the problems of implementation.[1]

What is hospital reimbursement attempting to achieve? The primary economics concern is efficiency, although other concerns can be incorporated such as macroeconomic expenditure control and equity. Here the traditional

---

[1] The local context is that of the UK and although policy implications from other environments will be drawn on, effort has been made to constrain empirical evidence, such as there is, to that gained from the UK.

Advances in Health Economics. Edited by Anthony Scott, Alan Maynard and Robert Elliott.
© 2003 John Wiley & Sons, Ltd

welfare approach is taken; efficiency is pursued through maximizing a welfare function normally defined as the sum of consumers' surplus and producers' surplus. Efficiency is thus linked to market outcomes. Such outcomes are difficult to replicate in the hospital sector. Notwithstanding these problems efficiency requires the pursuit of cost minimization subject to quality/outcome constraints, which in turn requires knowledge of production and cost relations. Building on this knowledge, prices must be linked to costs of production in such a way that incentives are created that move hospital outputs towards efficient levels. This can be done through ensuring that prices and costs are set at an efficient level. In turn this can be achieved through regulation or increasing competition. Both are possible in the hospital sector, but neither is easy to implement.

It may seem peculiar to consider prices in the hospital sector, particularly as most UK hospitals are publicly owned and managed. Since the introduction of the internal market however hospital prices (tariffs) are set for various individual treatment packages based on health care-related groupings which are the UK equivalent to diagnostic-related groups (DRGs). Information on the relationship between prices and costs gives some indication of the degree of market power enjoyed by individual hospitals. Information on the production and cost structure provides knowledge on the relative efficiency of hospital operation. This chapter begins by setting a benchmark against which efficiency may be defined. Essentially this entails outlining the conditions which support efficient price and cost structures. As will be noted, marginal or long-run average cost pricing becomes the standard. The difficulties of imposing such pricing rules on the hospital sector are then discussed – essentially these arise through problems in specifying production and cost relations. Then various incentive models of the sector are analysed. Following this there is some discussion of the impact of competition on NHS hospitals.

EFFICIENCY AND PRICING AND COST RULES

As an economic organization the hospital pursues production of the optimal mix of outputs at the socially efficient price.[2] If the allocation process is not efficient some resources are wasted and some patients will not be treated optimally. With a perfectly operating market, resources are moved to their highest valued use. For demand to operate efficiently the consumer must have perfect information over preferences and prices, maximize utility in a rational manner and have no influence over the price-setting process. This does not characterize the hospital sector.

---

[2] The question of what is meant by hospital output is considered later in the chapter. Ultimately it may be health outcome, at an intermediate level it may be a treated case.

On the supply side there are also problems. The main supply-side organization at the micro-level responsible for the efficiency of production decisions is the firm. The individual firm is seen traditionally to have a single owner pursuing profit maximization. At the highest abstract level the definition of efficiency employed is compatible with the perfectly competitive market structure. That is, for supply to operate efficiently it is sufficient (but not necessary) to have a perfectly competitive market dictate the behaviour of firms.

In the simple model of perfect competition individual firms operate within an industry characterized by certain assumptions. If these hold price equals average revenue and marginal revenue in the short and long run $(P = AR = MR)$; marginal revenue equals marginal cost in the short run and long run; and long-run output is uniquely determined where average cost equals marginal cost at the minimum of average cost. Price equals marginal cost $(P = MC)$ in the short and long run, and price is equal to marginal cost and average cost $(P = MC = AC)$ in the long run. These *price rules* determine optimal output. Equilibrium is stable; under perfect competition equilibrium is restored even if there is a *disturbance* to the market.

The perfectly competitive outcome has wide application in the real world as a benchmark that can be used by regulators against which efficiency can be calibrated when markets fail. In a number of regulated sectors the pricing rules stipulate that prices should be set equal to marginal cost or long-run average cost. In the utilities sector (for example the gas, electricity and telecommunications sectors) the basis of pricing can still be traced to these pricing rules (cf. Armstrong *et al.* 1994; Vickers & Yarrow 1998). If efficiency is the over-riding objective the pricing rules are such that price moves towards marginal cost or long-run average cost.

THE HOSPITAL AS A FIRM

It is widely acknowledged that market failures in the hospital sector are so extensive that efficiency will not evolve naturally (McGuire *et al.* 1991). Moreover the hospital does not fit easily into the notion of an individual economic firm. The objective may not be profit maximization. However the pursuit of non-profit maximization objectives may be operationally the same, surplus is maximized, and if efficiency is an over-riding concern any non-profit objective will be consistent with cost minimization. Secondly, it is difficult to specify a single owner/manager. Typically there are many actors within the hospital making decisions who might be characterized as clinicians or administrators. While a number of models of hospital behaviour have been suggested covering income maximizing through to quality/quantity maximizers, few have reconciled their conceptual model with the internal hospital production structure (Newhouse 1970; Pauly & Redisch 1973). One model that does has been proposed by Harris (1977).

This model emphasizes the internal resource allocation problem of the hospital, stating that the smooth production/cost conditions which characterize a traditional economic firm break down and the hospital is best viewed as two firms in one; the administrative functions and the medical functions. Each of these functions is locked into an allocation problem where resources have to be moved to their highest valued use, but where the price mechanism cannot solve the problem. Other mechanisms are therefore used including command structures (hierarchies) and co-operative or non-co-operative bargaining.

Harris (1977) recognizes that it is difficult to store hospital output – it must be produced on demand and is poorly substitutable across individual consumers (patients). Spot markets dominate and numerous idiosyncrasies of delivery dominate production. Hospital production is seen as a sequence of acquiring more information on diagnosis by the agent/clinician then providing more individual tailored treatments. The hospital responds to patient (agent) demands through a complicated series of bargaining processes. Spot market re-contracting is not adaptable enough to respond to these allocation problems. Given the potential uncertainty with each case, small number problems with the associated lack of competition fail to ensure clearing/equilibrium takes place. Moreover contractual re-negotiation would entail large transactions costs.

A number of conclusions arise from the recognition of the market within which the hospital operates and the importance of the production structure. First, the incentive structures facing the hospital and the agents within the hospital are critical to efficiency being achieved. Second, supply needs to be assured, as this is the cost of holding spare capacity for instantaneous demands. Hospitals may therefore be in deceptive equilibriums when there are cost over-runs or spare capacity. That is, given the complexity and uncertainty surrounding hospital production, the required availability of specialist services and the large costs (both private and social) in failing to respond instantaneously (or at least quickly) to specific demands pushes hospital production to be stochastic. Observed cost over-runs and spare capacity associated with any given hospital are consistent with this stochastic production process.

While this model does address the issue of the internal allocation process and the problems involved, and therefore helps explain the production and internal cost process, it says little about the reimbursement mechanisms or the optimal incentive structures that could be implemented under such circumstances. Neither does it formalize the nature of the stochastic production process. Both these issues are considered below, beginning with a general discussion of the hospital's production/cost relations.

HOSPITAL PRODUCTION AND COST RELATIONS

A number of problems exist in applying standard production theory to the hospital sector. First, the appropriate output measure must be defined. At least four measures have been suggested: an index of services provided; cases treated; number of successful treatments; and a measure of change in population health (Feldstein 1967). Demand is normally assumed to be exogenous, that is arrived at independently from the supply decisions affecting output level. This is not true in the hospital sector where demand is managed through the admission and discharge procedures. Output, however defined, is therefore not constrained by demand.

Hospital cost studies have concentrated on the first two definitions of hospital output given above, but even here there are problems. Take the number of treated cases, here we must control for type of illness, severity of illness, stage of illness, concomitant disease and patient characteristics which may aid recovery. Some of these issues have been addressed by the definition of DRGs in the USA and elsewhere.[3]

Neither is the relationship between hospital inputs well understood. The production function is not a fixed coefficients production function but is stochastic to some degree. Moreover, the appropriate technology may not be well defined or known – i.e. the appropriate functional relationship [the f in $Q = f(K,L)$] may be difficult to specify. Some have argued that health care technology is not, as conventionally assumed, exogenous (i.e. determined independently of the production process), but reacts to the third-party payment system that predominates in the sector (Weisbrod 1991). Also productivity is largely measured with regards to intermediate output, cases treated for example. It is difficult to verify the impact of greater input effort on final health outcome. On the input side labour is heterogeneous. Moreover it is difficult to define truly variable inputs – agency nursing is a clear example, but after this the distinction between fixed and variable inputs tends to merge. Short-run and long-run production relations are therefore difficult to define.

SCALE, CAPACITY AND STOCHASTIC DEMAND

Given these problems it is difficult to determine the efficient size of a hospital. The textbook defines optimal capacity as that consistent with economies of scale (i.e. minimum of LRAC). Suppose there is an assumed cost function, following Berki (1972) as drawn in Figure 7.1.

---

[3] These are groups of diseases based on an aggregation of the diseases classified by the International Classification of Disease (ICD) codes into 81 basic groups which are deemed to have similar resource requirements – although for Medicare reimbursement purposes, for instance, these are refined into over 400 separate groupings.

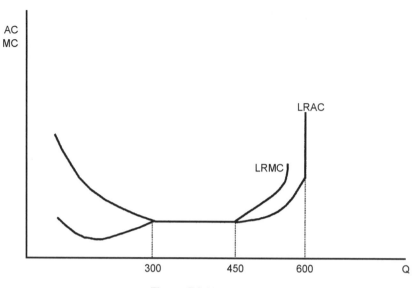

Figure 7.1 Hospital costs

Average cost reaches a minimum at 300 cases per unit of time, remains at this minimum up to 450 cases, increases gradually until 600 cases where it becomes infinite. No more than 600 cases can be produced regardless – this is absolute capacity. Output can be increased between 300 and 450 cases at constant cost (here $AC = MC$); so efficient capacity lies between 300 and 450 cases. What is the appropriate efficient capacity?

The hospital could set production at 450 cases, but if demand does not materialize then it is left with unused capacity. It could set production at 300, but if demand is above this level then some patients would not receive care, revenue would be lower than the achievable level (if reimbursement is related to cases treated) and reputation may suffer as patients are turned away. If demand is stochastic (i.e. uncertain) then the efficient level of output occurs where there is the optimal trade-off between not meeting demand and leaving capacity unused.

The determination of optimal capacity itself depends, again, on an appropriate specification of output. The precise stochastic nature of demand will vary according to the type of case being serviced. Hospitals distinguish between various forms of demand, for example elective and emergency admissions, with the former being controllable by the hospital, and the latter truly stochastic. This stochastic element can be a substantial proportion of overall demand. Bagust et al. (1999) estimated that emergency admissions now occupy 65% of available staffed beds in the UK.

Production responses to demand uncertainty are clearly important. Uncertainty results in a probability that the hospital faces unused resources after committing resources to the potential servicing of stochastic (e.g. emergency) demand, or under-commits and faces an excess demand for emergency care. In observing *ex post* unused capacity, standard analysis would suggest that the hospital is not operating efficiently. This does not, however, recognize an efficient production response to demand uncertainty.

Reserve capacity is held to service potential emergency demands. The hospital chooses how much of its total capacity to allocate to emergency demand based on its expectation of that demand. The expected number of patients treated is determined by the probability distribution of demand and the level at which the hospital chooses capacity. Mathematically, the expected number of emergencies treated is the mean to the left of the probability distribution truncated at the capacity constraint (i.e. number of emergency beds chosen). This is represented by:

$$\int_0^{q_{em}} x f(x) \mathrm{d}x + \int_{q_{em}}^{\infty} q_{em} f(x) \mathrm{d}x \tag{7.1}$$

where q_{em} is the level of capacity chosen on the efficient production envelope to service emergency (i.e. uncertain) demand, and the sum of the expression in equation (7.1) represents the expected level of demand. Hospitals choose the capacity level that services q_{em}. Each allocation of capacity to service emergency demand represents a point on this distribution and it is, therefore, possible to calculate the expected number of emergency admissions to be serviced for every capacity allocation.

Reserve capacity will be held by the hospital given that elective admission decisions are assumed entirely endogenous. Reserve capacity is, therefore, entirely dependent on the hospital's expectations of emergency demands. The actual capacity used will reflect the *ex post* realization of emergency demand. If realized demand differs from the expected level of demand hospital capacity may be too high or too low and, *ex post*, even after adjusting for uncertainty, costs will be imposed on the hospital.

As Chambers and Quiggin (2000) outline, it is important to recognize that the producer's goal is not to minimize the cost of producing a given *ex post* output, but to minimize the cost of producing a given *expected* level of output. In other words, efficiency is defined with regards to the production response to stochastic demand.

Estimates of hospital scale economies cannot be obtained without explicitly modelling the hospital's problem of maintaining sufficient standby capacity in the face of uncertain demand (Gaynor & Anderson 1995). Moreover economies of scope and integration with other parts of the health care sector are also important.

EMPIRICAL ESTIMATES OF COST FUNCTIONS

Given these difficulties it is not surprising that there has been widespread disagreement in the findings of the large body of empirical work on hospital cost functions. First the actual functional form must be specified. All agree that costs relate to output; but the devil is in the detail. A number of studies have used a flexible form approach. However, it should be noted that the most commonly estimated flexible form, the translog function, cannot deal with zero levels of output, due to the logarithmic aspect of the specification. If some hospitals in the sample population do not provide emergency or day case output they have to be excluded. Moreover, it is a mistaken interpretation of flexible functional forms to assume that they are approximating the true underlying technology. Estimation always requires some specification of functional form. The advantage of utilizing fully flexible functional forms is that they place few restrictions on the underlying technological structure, but at the cost of not necessarily providing truly global approximations, and imposing strong assumptions with regards to separability. An alternative way of proceeding would be through the use of Box–Cox transforms (Greene 1993).

The question remains, precisely how do costs relate to output? Different studies have considered different exact relationships – few have considered the endogenous nature of demand and/or the production reactions to stochastic demand (Gaynor & Anderson 1995; Carey 1996). Moreover most have used the volume of beds as a measure of scale. Given that this can be defined as a capital input rather than an output this may be a misspecification. This measure is used however as output is normally associated with short-term throughput of patients and is held to give a better indication of long-term output plans (Granneman et al. 1986).

Those who have reviewed the literature find that there are conflicting conclusions (see Granneman et al. 1986; Breyer 1987; Vita 1990; Ferguson et al. 1999). Cowing et al. (1983) review the early literature which is acknowledged to be based on ad hoc specifications but suggests that economies of scale do hold for small-sized hospitals but not for larger hospitals, defined as having more than 200 beds. The later, and in general more theoretically based literature is equivocal. Moreover to the extent that larger hospitals tend to treat the more complex cases and have greater depth or scope of production which tends to include specialized services, and both these characteristics tend to increase costs, this will bias the observation of economies of scale downwards. Thus there is no general conclusion reached on economies of scale (see Gaynor & Vogt 2000) or even the exact relation between hospital cost and output. As they point out there are large discrepancies in how the empirical literature has measured hospital output, a point consistent with the discussion on defining hospital output above.

REIMBURSEMENT ISSUES

Hospital revenue is generally received through a third party. The appropriate level of reimbursement requires some form of price and price–cost margin to be specified. The hospital will generally have better information over its production levels than the purchaser, thus there is a general observability and verification issue. The issue of the appropriate operating capacity given stochastic demand merely muddies the view further. Indeed the spare capacity issue can also be thought of from the insurer's perspective as one of attempting to guarantee supply assurance to cover the requirements of their insured population; hospital services must be on hand when required.

Reimbursing total hospital costs creates no incentive to minimize costs. Such a reimbursement mechanism will encounter technical inefficiency – the quantity of care supplied will be greater than is optimal – as well as productive inefficiency – quality may be higher than optimal. Cost-saving measures are unlikely to be introduced. That said reimbursement must be related to the costs of production in some manner. A typical scheme reimburses costs through the following general approach:

$$R = a + bC \qquad (7.2)$$

where R is the reimbursement revenue, a is a fixed fee and b represents a proportion of the costs (C) reimbursed. Two extremes exist. First, there is the cost plus fixed fee or cost-plus contract $(b = 1)$. The hospital is fully reimbursed. This creates low-level incentives. Alternatively, there is the fixed-price contract $(b = 0)$. The hospital is responsible for and recipient of all cost savings. No costs are reimbursed, only a fee is paid creating a high-powered incentive. Incentive contracts based on this linear relationship (where b has a slope of between 0 and 1) share the degree of risk taken by the hospital and the purchaser. Ideally costs have to be observable and possibly some notion of minimum cost defined. Given the difficulty in specifying the production/cost relationship, specification of the optimal reimbursement level is problematic.

INCENTIVES

In any hospital sector approximately 70% of expenditure is tied to labour and it is therefore obvious that the analysis of pay structures (or more generally reimbursement structures) to ensure efficient performance of labour ought to be an important topic. It is therefore perhaps surprising that relatively little attention has been given to this area. More so given that issues of unobservability and non-verifiability abound in this sector.

In the health care sector a principal (patient) employs an agent (doctor) to work for them. This situation is complicated by the fact that the doctor can also be seen as an agent for another principal (the purchaser; whether this is an insurance company or the government). The principal (in our case the purchaser or patient) may not be able to fully observe or verify the agent's (health care provider's) actions. The outcome of an agent's actions may well be observed, but the relationship between the agent's actions and the observed outcome are stochastic. An agent's actions do not fully determine the observed outcome. Under such circumstances the principal must design the reimbursement package in such a way that it indirectly gives the appropriate incentive to the agent to undertake those actions which are compatible with an efficient outcome.

A major problem arising in this area is moral hazard; agents may have better information than the principal over their performance. In particular unobservable behaviour/hidden actions may be present. Here are two examples. A doctor may not operate as a perfect agent for his patient. If the doctor were a perfect agent for the patient alone then they would have identical objectives to those of the patient; but the doctor may have his own goals either to increase his income or to maintain resource use for his own benefit rather than the patient's (he may have a research agenda, or be holding on to scarce resources to empire build, or to secure these resources for future use). It is difficult for the patient to observe this behaviour and therefore to assess whether the doctor is behaving efficiently or not. A second major problem is patient selection and cream-skimming; costs are reduced through accepting low-risk patients.

In both cases it will be difficult to specify the optimal reimbursement to ensure that the most efficient outcome is attained. Health care providers may not work with optimal effort. A central feature is that the agent does not bear the full consequences of his own actions, as the principal bears some cost, either in real terms through lack of optimal treatment or in financial terms through inefficient health care delivery.

Shliefer (1985) considers the issue of optimal reimbursement when the purchaser/regulator does not know the precise costs of production. Medicare hospitals are used as an example of regulatory asymmetry of information over costs. The model assumes constant marginal costs of production (c_0), which the firm can reduce to c by investing in $R(c)$ on cost-reducing efforts. $R(c_0) = 0$ and the rate of change of cost-reducing investment is negative [i.e. $R'(c) < 0$].

The surplus (V) generated by the hospital is:

$$V = (p - c)\, q(p) + T - R(c) \qquad (7.3)$$

where p is the unit price, q is the quantity of health care produced and T is a lump-sum transfer made to the firm. With no information asymmetries the regulator would pick c, p and T to maximize the sum of consumer surplus and hospital surplus subject to a breakeven constraint ($V \geqslant 0$).

The solution is gained by examining:

$$\int q(x)\delta x + (p - c)\, q(p) + T - R(c) \tag{7.4}$$

with c chosen such that:

$$-R'(c^*) = q(p^*) \tag{7.5}$$

with $p^* = c^*$ and $R(c^*) = T^*$.

These conditions merely state that we are dealing with cost-minimizing conditions for producing output q. They are given by differentiating equation (7.3) with respect to c and setting equal to 0. The intuition is that, given price equals total marginal costs of production and effort (i.e. $p = c^*$), the hospital will invest in cost-reducing technology until the incremental (marginal) investment cost $R'(c)$ equals the incremental saving in production cost $q(c^*)$, where given $p = c^*$ the incremental saving in production cost is $-q'(p^*)$. $R = T$ is merely a breakeven condition. Investment in cost-reducing technology is declining [$R'(c) < 0$], so average cost is always declining as the variable cost of production is constant and there is a fixed cost equal to R. If $p = $ total MC then a transfer of R is necessary to breakeven. So p^* and T^* results in the first-best outcome. If the regulator states that p can equal whatever c the hospital specifies and T is set to whatever R is set by the hospital then the optimal will not be achieved. Moreover, because of asymmetric information the regulator cannot observe R^* and c^*.

Shleifer shows that the first best can be achieved under a weaker condition; if the regulator sets p equal to the average observed costs among other identical hospitals in the market and R equal to the average investment R for other identical hospitals. The basic idea works as follows. If total revenue for each hospital is set equal to the average cost for the sample of hospitals, this gives an incentive to each hospital to cut costs to below the average, through increasing their investment in cost-reducing technology, to generate a surplus. When all hospitals do this the average cost falls and this incentive continues until price is equal to c^*. With price set to the optimal level (i.e. equal to c^*) some hospitals will of course have to receive T^*. As long as there is no collusion and the sample of identical hospitals is large there is little loss from simply setting price equal to the average across all hospitals. Shliefer also considers the case when no transfers are allowed and shows that prospective payment based on observed average cost is second best. So he shows that a fixed pricing rule based on observable data can lead hospitals to efficient production. If, for example, DRGs are defined based on average costs he states that prospective pricing is close to optimal.

Another way of considering the performance is to look not at surplus-maximizing hospitals, but at the reimbursement of hospitals who employ utility-maximizing clinicians. Here the clinician is operating as an agent for both hospital and patient. A starting point for this type of analysis is the paper by Ellis and McGuire (1986). In their model the patient is not charged for health care (q). A benefit function is specified [$B(q)$]. The patient's clinician derives utility in two ways; from the surplus generated by the hospital and from patient satisfaction:

$$U(\pi^h, B) \tag{7.6}$$

where $\pi^h(q) = R(q) - c^h q$. This is merely revenue minus cost, with c^h the marginal cost of producing health care which is held constant.

Clinician's choice of q satisfies:

$$\frac{dU}{d\pi^h}\frac{d\pi^h}{dq} + \frac{dU}{dB}\frac{dB}{dq} = 0 \tag{7.7}$$

Rearranging gives:

$$\pi^h = -\text{MRS}_{\pi,B}\frac{dB}{dq} \tag{7.8}$$

as the marginal rate of substitution between hospital profit and patient benefit for the clinician is defined as:

$$\text{MRS}_{\pi,B} = \frac{dU/dB}{dU/d\pi^h} > 0$$

Thus in equilibrium the clinician will choose to equate hospital and patient marginal benefits, having adjusted for the subjective rate at which he is willing to trade these off.

Having set up this equilibrium the effect of three different reimbursement rules on this optimum are considered from a private perspective (i.e. $dB/dq > / < 0$) and a welfare perspective (i.e. $dB/dq > / < c^h > 0$). Consider full cost reimbursement. Revenue always covers costs (i.e. $d\pi^h/dq = 0$). From equation (7.7) $dB/dq = 0$, implying that the clinician supplies the patient with the (private) optimal quantity of health care. But this must also mean that the welfare solution is non-optimal and there is an over-supply of health care since $dB/dq = 0 < c^h$.

Under prospective reimbursement the hospital receives, say, G for the treatment of the patient. So $\pi^h = G - c^h q$ and $d\pi^h/dq = -c^h < 0$. From equation (7.7) $db/dq > 0$ so the patient is receiving less health care than under full cost reimbursement, as the marginal cost of producing q is fully incurred by the hospital. Social efficiency on the other hand may be achieved, but only when the MRS $= 1$, that is when the clinician is a perfect agent (defined as having an equal weight on both the hospital and patient benefit functions).

With cost sharing the hospital is reimbursed a fraction $\gamma \in [0,1]$ of the marginal cost of health care treatment and the hospital bears the rest of the reimbursement. So $\pi^h = G + (\gamma - 1)c^h q$. Setting $\gamma = (1 - \mathrm{MRS}_{\pi,B})$ generates $dB/dq = c^h$ (which is the social optimum; i.e. where marginal benefits = marginal cost). This forces the clinician (through the hospital) to bear more costs than full reimbursement, but less than prospective payment; γ leads to optimal production of q. Of course if $\gamma = 0$ prospective payment is returned.

The Ellis and McGuire model provides a simple, linear incentive model showing that full cost reimbursement leads to over-supply of health care and prospective payment leads to under-supply. The basic mechanism for these results is that the patient has no role in the decision-making, the clinician takes all consumption decisions, and patients are fully insured. With full cost reimbursement neither the patient nor the purchaser constrains the health care provider from raising the quantity of treatment, while with fixed fee payment such a constraint will be binding. The model is therefore consistent with the earlier discussion of low and high-powered incentives.

The Ellis and McGuire model considers incentive contracts as they relate to the quantity of treatment produced, but does not consider effort or quality explicitly. Ma (1994), amongst others, introduces quality dimensions into the incentive contract. The fundamental assumption in all such models is that demand reacts to increasing quality provision. Under this assumption the general conclusion is that prospective payment provides the optimal levels of effort while cost reimbursement leads to an over-supply of quality-enhancing effort. The basic intuition is that with cost reimbursement the hospital can increase effort in the quality dimension as it gets fully reimbursed for this. As it attracts more patients (demand is linked to quality remember) the hospital gains a payment of some fixed amount per patient. With prospective payment the incentive is to move to the optimal level of effort in quality and cost-reducing technology as specified by the regulator's first best.

Like most models this conclusion reflects the assumptions. In this case that demand is price-inelastic due to the full coverage of health care insurance, and this leads to efficiency being achieved by the regulator setting a single price for the hospital. With price elasticity, introduced through some co-insurance schedule, non-linear reimbursement would be necessary (i.e. some mix of cost reimbursement and prospective payment).

Chalkey and Malcolmson (1998) apply a similar model to the NHS. The health care provider has a benefit function $b(x,q)$ which is the number of patients treated (x) with quality (q). The cost of treatment $c(x,q,e)$ is related to the number treated with quality (q) as well as the effort (e) the hospital invests in keeping costs down. The hospital receives direct utility $s - v(x,q,e)$, where s is the financial surplus and $v(\cdot)$ is the disutility of providing services, assumed to be increasing in e.

The purchaser's objective is to maximize:

$$b(x,q) + s - v(x,q,e) - (1 + \alpha)[c(x,q,e) + s] \qquad (7.9)$$

Thus the objective relates to consumer benefits plus hospital utility minus costs [weighted $(1 + \alpha)$ by tax costs]. This objective is maximized subject to two constraints. A capacity constraint $[x \leqslant x'(q)]$ and a reservation utility constraint $[s - v(x,q,e) \geqslant v']$ which gives the minimum utility for which the hospital will accept a contract. With substitution and noting the second constraint becomes an equality if $\alpha > 0$, we have the purchaser's first-best outcome specified as:

$$\max b(x,q) - (1 + \alpha)[c(x,q,e) - \alpha v'] \qquad (7.10)$$

The first-best outcome (x^*,q^*,e^*) can be found by differentiating equation (7.10) with respect to x, q and e.

The hospital, on the other hand, maximizes:

$$s - v(x,q,e) \qquad (7.11)$$

subject to a capacity constraint $[x > x'(q)]$ and the budget constraint $\{B[x,n(q),c(x,q,e)] - c(x,q,e) - s\}$. On substitution we have:

$$\max B[x,n(q),c(x,q,e)] - c(x,q,e) - v(x,q,e) \qquad (7.12)$$

It is difficult to achieve first-best outcomes here as the purchaser has a small number of instruments to cover the policy targets and consequently the outcome achieved depends on the number of quality dimensions which are pursued, and the relationship between demand $[n(q)]$ and benefit $[b(x,q)]$. That said, Chalkey and Malcolmson replicate Ma's (1994) solution, over one dimension of quality within a demand-constrained situation. The intuition behind this result is that the hospital can increase revenue through increasing demand, and it can increase demand by increasing quality of care. Quality of care will be increased to any level the purchaser is willing to fund.

This result only holds if demand is constrained. If demand is unconstrained treatment goes beyond the optimal number in order to achieve first-best quality. If capacity is constrained, the hospital does not have the capacity to treat all those demanding health care at optimal quality levels, so quality is produced below optimal levels. To resolve this a mixed payment (lump sum transfer plus a fixed price per treated patient) is required. The intuition is that hospitals will offer higher quality to attract patients, if payment is given for increasing demand, even if all patients are not treated.

They then consider multidimensional quality aspects, noting that the number of instruments may be too small for the dimensions of quality that the purchaser is attempting to manipulate. If quality in any one dimension of health care increases demand relative to purchaser benefit in the same proportion as any other increase from a different quality dimension, then a mixed payment system will produce an efficient outcome (the optimal levels of benefit, quality and effort will be achieved). This is the case as the mixed price is inducing quality responses in an equiproportional manner across the different dimensions as demand changes.

The importance of this result is that it shows that if patients and purchasers have the same relative valuations of different dimensions of quality of care a mixed payment system can attain efficiency. In the model the patient must recognize quality, the hospitals must have well-defined utility functions (objectives) and the cost of treatment functions must be known.

This model raises the importance of quality as a determinant of optimal reimbursement in the hospital sector. Indeed as Dranove and Satterthwaite (2000) suggest price and quality interaction may be critical in determining output levels in the hospital sector. Again assuming the purchasers have incomplete information over cost and quality levels they show that, against a general background of poor purchaser knowledge and product differentiation (i.e. a monopolistic market), quality may be excessive if price elasticity is low, or too low if quality elasticity is low and purchasers are price-sensitive. Note also that price will be above marginal cost of any given level of quality production as dictated by the monopsonistic market assumption. Even if quality is fully observed, say published hospital death rates (currently advocated as a marker of quality in the UK) do fully correlate with hospital quality, if price/cost conditions are not fully observable this can still lead to price–cost margins being excessive, resulting in the over-production of quality.

HOSPITAL COMPETITION AND REGULATION

In pursuing efficiency benchmarks, such as the pricing rule gained from perfectly competitive markets (i.e. $P = MC = AC$), may be used. Given that the consumer is particularly lacking in the information required to specify demand, third-party payment is the norm and increasing returns to specialization characterize the hospital sector. Even if heavily regulated competition led by patient demand is unlikely to be successful. Thus while markets do exist in a number of countries the interaction is always based on higher levels of aggregation. Purchasers, acting as agents for patients, are held to have better knowledge of the market operation due to longer-term purchasing relationships. However they may well have their own objectives and may not represent their population's preferences properly.

Turning to providers, market-based solutions are argued to encourage price competition, thereby ensuring costs are minimized in a market where verification of delivered service is difficult. Nonetheless market competition may be limited as information on the quality of health care provision may be weak. Indeed, if there is incomplete information on provider quality then prices may act in a perverse manner to signal quality levels – higher average costs and therefore prices may be taken to represent higher quality (Stiglitz 1987).

Moreover capacity constraints may distort competition as the purchasers of health care may seek to assure themselves of some part of supply. Purchasers may overestimate the capacity constraints they face and pay, in advance, for unutilized health care. This is the argument forwarded by Fenn et al. (1994) in explaining the dominance of block contracting, where hospitals provide access to their capacity in exchange for a lump sum prospective payment. When provider capacity is constrained the purchaser may be prepared to pay a premium to secure such capacity for their population in the form of a block contract. Obviously as capacity grows this incentive is weakened. The irony of increased competition is that in the short run it may lead to capacity reductions, which increases the incentive to secure supply. Such incentives promote the desire to foster long-term relationships, which typify most markets in reality, as part of the attempt to assure access to provider facilities when demand occurs.

Fenn et al. (1994) assume the purchaser commits to pay a prospective payment (e.g. a block contract). This payment is enough to cover fixed costs (F), variable costs (c), which are defined over N, the numbers treated, q, the quality of care and supplier effort, e, such that $c(N,q,e)$ and non-monetary costs which capture the direct utility effects of N, q and e [say $v(N,q,e)$]. So the prospective payment is:

$$R = F + c(\cdot) + v(\cdot) \tag{7.13}$$

The purchaser then considers the increase in cost of having an additional patient treated above the supply assured level (N). That is, what does it cost the purchaser if they go beyond the supply assured level? This cost is presumed higher because of the higher transactions costs incurred in seeking out alternative providers.

The purchaser then has a trade-off. The purchaser could increase the size of its contract to the provider (i.e. increase the contracted N) which would ensure that if more treatments were required they would be provided at the lower contracted price but in doing so, of course, they may be locking into more than the number of treatments necessary to service their population.

This problem is made more difficult when the demand for treatments is uncertain. With demand for treatments specified as a random variable x with density function $g(x)$ and distribution function $G(x)$ then the purchasers choose N to minimize cost through:

$$\min_{N} c(N,q^*,e^*) + v(N,q^*,e^*) + \frac{\int_{N}^{\infty} xg(x)\partial x}{1 - G(N)} \qquad (7.14)$$

Costs are minimized where the purchaser commits to some N^* greater than the lowest level of demand.

If supply assurance is an issue purchasers will attempt to utilize any monopsonistic power to move providers to accept prospective payment contracts that resemble block contracts and a higher proportion of providers' revenue will become fixed rather than variable. Csaba and Fenn (1997), noting the predominance of block contracting in the UK, tested the hypothesis of supply assurance using data from 71 NHS Hospital Trusts to calculate the proportion of their contractual revenue that was volume-related or fixed. The results of this study tended to confirm that block contracts were more likely where there are capacity constraints, as in the NHS.

The issue of bargaining power with regards to providers and purchasers in the UK was analysed by Propper (1996). A simple pricing algorithm is used to consider the degree of market power wielded by individual providers (NHS Hospital Trusts) where

$$P = (1 + 1/\eta)c \qquad (7.15)$$

with P equal to price, c equal to marginal cost (although in the event proxied by average cost) and $(1 + 1/\eta)$ is the mark-up of price over cost which is a function of competition, bargaining power and some other factors (including hospital characteristics). The hypothesis that price was determined solely by cost of production was tested across four hospital specialties. It was found that prices were not solely related to cost and there was weak evidence that market conditions had the expected impacts on price; that is the stronger the implied competition and the weaker the bargaining power, the lower the price.[4]

In related work, which considered the hospital as an entity but controlled for case mix, Csaba (1995) tested a number of hypotheses concerning the determination of average costs. The explanatory variables included measures

---

[4] There is a large US-dominated literature on the relationship between hospital costs and price competition. Generally this relationship will reflect to some degree the actual market structure (i.e. the market structure helps determine the price–cost mark-up). In this chapter the UK findings are highlighted. The reader interested in the more general literature is directed to the reviews by Dranove and Satterthwaite (2000), Sloan (2000), Gaynor and Vogt (2000) and Salkever (2000). If a general conclusion can be reached from this vast literature it is that competition does have an impact; the size of the impact is disputed.

of output based on finished consultant episodes, case mix, technology, factor input prices and a number of market structure control variables. The findings were mixed. The higher the concentration of purchasers' power in the internal market the lower was provider cost, implying that purchasers can influence the efficiency of provider units. There was weak support consistent with the competitive behaviour of hospitals being linked to market structure – i.e. the more competitive the market the lower the cost. This is in accordance with Soderlund *et al.* (1996) who found that the considerable variation in hospital costs could be explained through variation in the outputs produced and wage and property costs. They also found that trust status and increased purchasing power were associated with lower hospital costs, although hospital market share had no impact on cost. Csaba (1997), in a different specification, found some support for the hypothesis that competition did lower cost, however.

All of these UK studies were undertaken during a time when the internal market was regulated. While hospitals were apparently allowed to retain financial surpluses, borrow capital funds and set local pay and conditions the market conditions governing these were tightly regulated. NHS hospitals were required to break even, capital market access was restricted through centrally imposed rates of return and, most importantly, after allowing for capital adjustments prices were set equal to average cost. As Propper *et al.* (1998) note, such a regulatory framework makes the hospital vulnerable to short-run changes in income thereby providing an incentive to break the regulatory requirement that price equals average cost. Where costs are joint and the apportionment of costs to any individual service is not clearly specified it is difficult to verify that the regulation is being maintained. Propper *et al.* test the hypothesis that the regulation is being upheld through use of a model similar to that in Propper (1996), testing the degree to which hospitals can mark-up above cost controlling for a number of confounding characteristics. Their results demonstrate that the regulatory rule ($P = AC$) is being broken.

The optimal level of capacity relates to long-term decisions of the potential growth for services facing any particular provider. To invest in additional capacity, however, providers must have access to capital funds. In other words, competition has both short and long-run effects and the full advantages are not reaped if both time horizons are not catered for. If short-run average cost is falling merely because of output expansion, rather than competition, sooner or later capacity constraints will be met. A demand for new capacity will arise, but if new capital funds are not forthcoming output will face physical constraints and, eventually, short-run average costs will rise reflecting diminishing returns. Competition may induce the desire to expand output in the short run, after all even in budget-constrained systems it is desirable to have patients if patients generate income.

CONCLUSIONS

What is known? Generally the efficiency benchmark is to move to a pricing rule which mimics perfect competition. That is, where price is equal to marginal cost, or to long-run average cost. The latter is more appropriate for example if there are increasing economies of scale – which depth of production, specialization and a political desire to respond quickly to stochastic (emergency) demand may enforce. Of course hospitals do not operate like simple profit-maximizing firms. Objectives differ. Production/cost relationships are 'fuzzy' and not straightforward. Optimal capacity is difficult to identify given stochastic demand for some services. Most hospitals have some degree of monopoly power. Under such conditions incentive payment schemes must be devised that recognize the observability and verification problems that exist in defining optimal hospital output levels in terms of both quality and quantity. Full cost reimbursement is inefficient. Prospective reimbursement with cost sharing is better. Even so it is difficult to identify appropriate incentive payment schemes over many levels of quality. Yardstick competition moves towards the optimal, if there is no gaming (e.g. collusion) by hospitals, and hospital product is not differentiated by, for example, quality. If contracts are to be specified in advance of purchase and capacity constraints exist supply assurance may follow.

Given that it is difficult to verify effort–output relations, observe optimal cost–quality relations and an inherent degree of cross-subsidization across services may exist any regulation is difficult to enforce. Empirical analysis of the hospital sector suggests that competition does lower costs, but the effect is muted. Moreover unless there is explicit consideration of quality, price competition may have adverse welfare effects particularly where costs are not easily observed. The present UK system is hoping to enforce competition through the impact of the purchasers of health care pursuing cost-minimizing policies and the enforcement of DRG-type pricing. If the hospital product is truly a differential one, differentiated through quality and resulting in a monopolistic market, the crude imposition of yardstick-based competition may lead to a general underproduction of quality if quality signals are difficult to observe and purchasers are cost-conscious. If hospitals are grouped inappropriately, driving down average costs through yardstick competition may simply reduce average quality of care. Even if grouped appropriately, squeezing hospitals' price–cost mark-ups may do nothing other than reduce quality of care, if quality is difficult to observe. Purchasers may have more knowledge of the quality signals than individual patients, but even this will be far from perfect. The optimal size of the purchasing unit becomes critical if repeat purchasing is the main mechanism in determining quality or monopsonistic power is relied on to constrain the monopolistic market structure within which the hospital operates.

ACKNOWLEDGEMENTS

We would like to acknowledge the helpful comments gained from Shelley Farrar, Bob Elliott, Alan Maynard and Tony Scott as well as the HERU conference participants generally. Liability for errors of commission and omission remain with the authors.

REFERENCES

Armstrong M, Cowan S and Vickers J (1994) *Regulatory Reform: Economic Analysis and British Experience*. MIT Press, Cambridge, MA.

Bagust A, Place M and Posnett J (1999) Dynamics of bed use in accommodating emergency admissions; stochastic simulation model. *British Medical Journal*, **319**, 155–158.

Berki S (1972) *Hospital Economics*. Lexington, Massachusetts.

Breyer F (1987) The specification of a hospital cost function: a comment on the recent literature. *Journal of Health Economics*, **6**, 147–157.

Carey K (1996) *Stochastic demand for hospitals and optimising "excess" bed capacity*. Discussion Paper, US Department of Veterans Affairs.

Chalkey M and Malcolmson J (1998) Contracting for health care with unmonitored quality. *Economic Journal*, **108**, 1093–1110.

Chambers R and Quiggin J (2000) *Uncertainty, Production, Choice and Agency*. Cambridge University Press, Cambridge.

Cowing T, Holtmann A and Powers S (1983) Hospital cost analysis: a survey and evaluation of recent studies. *Advances in Health Economics and Health Services Research*, **4**, 257–303.

Csaba I (1995) *Quasi-markets and the UK National Health Service*. Unpublished paper, Centre for Socio-Legal Studies, University of Oxford.

Csaba I (1997) *Quasi-markets and hospital behaviour, analysing the UK health reforms*. Paper presented to the Health Economists' Study Group conference.

Csaba I and Fenn P (1997) Contractual choice in the managed health care market. *Journal of Health Economics*, **16**, 579–588.

Dranove D and Satterthwaite M (2000) The industrial economics of health care markets. In AJ Culyer and J Newhouse (Eds), *The Handbook of Health Economics*. Elsevier, Amsterdam.

Ellis R and McGuire T (1986) Provider behaviour under prospective reimbursement. *Journal of Health Economics*, **5**, 129–151.

Feldstein M (1967) *Economic Analysis for Health Services Efficiency: Econometric Studies of the British NHS*. North-Holland, Amsterdam.

Fenn P, Rickman N and McGuire A (1994) Contracts and supply assurance in the UK health market. *Journal of Health Economics*, **13**, 125–144.

Ferguson B, Sheldon T and Posnett J (1999) *Concentration and Choice in Health Care*. Royal Society of Medicine Press, London.

Gaynor M and Anderson G (1995) Uncertain demand, the structure of hospital costs and the cost of an empty bed. *Journal of Health Economics*, **14**, 291–317.

Gaynor M and Vogt W (2000) Antitrust and competition in health care markets. In AJ Culyer and J Newhouse (Eds), *The Handbook of Health Economics*. Elsevier, Amsterdam.

Granneman T, Brown R and Pauly M (1986) Estimating hospital costs, a multiple output analysis. *Journal of Health Economics*, **5**, 107–127.

Greene WH (1993) *Econometric Analysis*. Prentice-Hall, New Jersey.

Harris J (1977) The internal organisation of the hospital: some economic implications. *Bell Journal of Economics*, **8**, 467–482.

Ma C (1994) Health care payment systems. *Journal of Economics and Management Strategy*, **3**, 93–112.

McGuire A, Fenn P and Mayhew K (1991) *Providing Health Care: The Economics of Alternative Systems of Finance and Delivery*. Oxford University Press, Oxford.

Newhouse J (1970) Towards a theory of nonprofit institutions: an economic model of the hospital. *American Economic Review*, **60**, 64–74.

Pauly M and Redisch M (1973) The not-for-profit hospital as a physicians' cooperative. *American Economic Review*, **63**, 87–99.

Propper C (1996) Market structure and prices: the responses of hospitals in the UK National Health Service to competition. *Journal of Public Economics*, **61**, 307–335.

Propper C, Wilson D and Soderlund N (1998) *The effects of regulation and competition in the NHS internal market*. Department of Economics Discussion Paper, University of Bristol.

Salkever D (2000) Regulation of prices and investment in hospitals in the US. In AJ Culyer and J Newhouse (Eds), *The Handbook of Health Economics*. Elsevier, Amsterdam.

Shliefer (1985) A theory of yardstick competition. *RAND Journal of Economics*, **16**, 319–327.

Sloan F (2000) Not-for-profit ownership and hospital behaviour. In AJ Culyer and J Newhouse (Eds), *The Handbook of Health Economics*. Elsevier, Amsterdam.

Soderlund N, Csaba I, Gray A, Milne R and Raftery J (1996) Impact of the NHS reforms on English hospital productivity: an analysis of the first three years. *British Medical Journal*, **315**, 1126–1129.

Stiglitz J (1987) Monopoly, non-linear pricing and imperfect information: the insurance market. *Review of Economic Studies*, **44**, 407–430.

Vickers J and Yarrow G (1998) *Privitisation: An Economic Analysis*. MIT, Cambridge, MA.

Vita M (1990) Exploring hospital production relations with flexible functional forms. *Journal of Health Economics*, **9**, 1–21.

Weisbrod B (1991) The health care quadrilemma: an essay on technological change, insurance, quality of care, and cost containment. *Journal of Economic Literature*, **29**, 523–552.

8

Measuring Efficiency in Dental Care

DAVID PARKIN
Department of Economics, City University, London

NANCY DEVLIN
Department of Economics, City University, London

INTRODUCTION: ORAL HEALTH AND DENTAL CARE AS ECONOMIC GOODS

In many respects, dental care is simply a specific service to which health economists have applied the same analytical tools also applied to other health care services. The market for dental care shares some of the same characteristics as health care generally, such as uncertainty and consumers' lack of knowledge. The challenges faced in economic analysis, such as the valuation of health outcomes, are also familiar. Yet there are also distinctive features of dental care markets.

Most notably, dental care has much less of a tradition of third-party involvement of any kind in funding, whether by insurance or government, than other types of health care. Out-of-pocket payments for dental care are common even in systems where most other types of health care are 'free'. There is also a greater reliance on private ownership of dental care delivery. These characteristics, in turn, may be explained by the 'special' nature of dental disease (see Box 8.1). Differing views on the importance of these factors – and on the importance attached to oral health and dental services in contributing to well-being and health – are reflected in the variety of arrangements that exist internationally to finance and provide dental care.

One of the consequences of these special characteristics is that the volume of economic analyses in dental care is limited. Sintonen and Linosmaa (2000) provide an overview of the literature. The Health Economics Research Unit at Aberdeen University has a long tradition of analyses of dental care, including

Advances in Health Economics. Edited by Anthony Scott, Alan Maynard and Robert Elliott.
© 2003 John Wiley & Sons, Ltd

Box 8.1 'Special' characteristics of dental disease and treatment

1. Dental disease is concentrated in a highly localized area of the anatomy; there are only two main dental diseases (caries and periodontal disease), both of which are extremely common and can be treated by a small range of well-established procedures.

2. Although, like ill health generally, dental illness is uncertain, the degree of uncertainty and its consequences are less than for other conditions. Maintenance needs (examinations, scaling, replacement fillings) can be predicted with reasonable accuracy and budgeted for – thus dental care is not an obvious candidate for private insurance. Such insurance arrangements as exist are more appropriately thought of as prepayment schemes, rather than insurance as such.

3. Dental disease is both continual and cumulative: consumers have been characterized as 'perpetual patients' in constant need of treatment (Cooper 1980). The greater familiarity of consumers with dental illness and treatment may mean they are better informed in their decisions regarding frequently consumed dental services than for medical services generally, and less prone to providers of care recommending excessive treatment. In most cases there is a simple (albeit radical), inexpensive substitute for more expensive, conservative treatment options: extraction.

4. Neither caries nor periodontal disease is infectious, so the presence of dental ill health and the consumption of dental care do not directly impose external effects on others.

5. With the exception of oral cancer, dental disease is not life-threatening. It can, if allowed to progress, cause considerable pain, but does not usually lead to serious permanent disabilities.

6. Dental illness rarely intrudes upon normal role obligations, and is increasingly concerned with cosmetic rather than functional considerations – hence the suggestion that it is comparable with other conditions relating primarily to personal comfort and appearance, such as obesity and baldness (Davis 1981).

Source: Devlin *et al.* (2002).

the production of dental care (Gray 1982); the need and demand for dental care and the role of prices (Yule 1984; Yule & Parkin 1985; Parkin & Yule 1988; Yule *et al.* 1988); the evaluation of dental services (Yule *et al.* 1986) and the financing and organization of dental services (Parkin & Yule 1986; Yule 1988). This chapter draws upon and extends these contributions to the literature.

This chapter focuses on two questions regarding the efficiency of dental care services at the 'micro' and 'macro' level respectively. First, to what extent can economic evaluation inform the efficient allocation of health care resources within and between dental care and other health care services? Second, given the various means by which dental care might be funded and delivered, what is the relative performance of alternative systems of funding and providing dental care in terms of the extent to which each results in improvements in oral health outcomes? In each case, the key issues are identified, the 'state of the play' in research reviewed and directions for future research suggested.

CHALLENGES IN THE ECONOMIC EVALUATION OF DENTAL CARE

The literature on the economic evaluation of dental services has two features. First, a limited number of economic evaluations have been published and those that have, with few exceptions, are rudimentary cost-effectiveness analyses that relate cost to a descriptive measure of dental health (for a survey, see Sintonen & Linosmaa 2000). While some cost–benefit analyses have been undertaken, these generally measure benefits only in terms of savings arising from interventions, underestimating the benefits to society (Yule *et al.* 1986). Second, the topics on which these evaluations have been performed tend to be on the margins of established public spending programmes (child dental care services; preventive dental services). This follows logically from the restricted role of collective funding in dental care services.

The most widely used outcome measure used in cost-effectiveness analyses – DMFT – is a simple count of affected teeth. There are important limitations with this as a measure of oral health for use in economic evaluation (Birch 1986) as it ignores changes to the *quality* of a tooth. For example, an individual who has one carious tooth requiring treatment has a score of '1' (decayed); when treated they have one filled tooth, which also counts as '1' (filled). Their total DMFT score remains unaltered, despite the change in the quality of the stock of teeth. The individual concerned is unlikely to be indifferent between the two states described.

In order to overcome this problem, Birch (1986) developed a measure for quality adjusted tooth years (QATYs). Possible tooth types are decayed (d), missing (m), filled (f) and sound (s). An individual's values for s and m are set at 1 and 0, with values sought for d and f, with the total value of the individual's dental stock at a given point in time equalling the sum of these values. The individual's lifetime QATYs are obtained by taking the sum over an individual's lifetime. A variant on this – expected QATYs – takes account of changes in oral health by incorporating probabilities of changed oral health states (Antczak-Bouckoms & Weinstein 1987). While QATYs are an improvement on simple, clinical measures, an important limitation is that they cover only caries-related problems and outcomes. Other, potentially relevant oral health states (e.g. orthodontic problems) are not included.

Perhaps the most notable feature of the literature on the economic evaluation of oral health has been the lack of progress, post-QATYs, in establishing valuations. The importance of measuring oral health-related quality of life (QoL), focusing on the *impact* of disease rather than the clinical presence of it, has increasingly been recognized by dental health researchers (Locker 1995), although this research does not appear to have been motivated or informed by the requirements of economic evaluation. Research has occasionally explored the impact of oral health problems on generic QoL measures for *overall* health, e.g. the Sickness Impact Profile (Reisine & Weber 1989) and the 15D (Arinen & Sintonen 1995), but more usually involves the development of quality of life measures specific to *oral* health. Examples include: the Dental Health Index (DHI) (Spolsky *et al.* 1983); the Dental Functional Status Index (Rosenberg *et al.* 1988); Socio-Dental Indicators (Cushing *et al.* 1986); General Oral Health Assessment Index (GOHAI) (Atchison & Dolan 1990); Subjective Oral Health Indicators (Locker 1995); Oral Health Impact Profile (OHIP) (Slade & Spencer 1994), later shortened to the OHIP14 (Slade 1997); the Dental Impacts on Daily Living (DIDL) (Leao & Sheiham 1996); and Oral Impacts on Daily Performance (OIDP) (Adulyanon *et al.* 1996). The most recent addition to this literature, the Oral Health Quality of Life-UK(W) [OHQoL-UK(W)] (McGrath & Bedi 2001), seeks individual's ratings of the impact of each dimension of oral health on quality of life; however, this is done by means of a five-point scale so does not directly facilitate quality of life weightings of the type that would facilitate economic evaluation. Many of the oral health QoL instruments generate sub-item scores that are weighted and summed to generate a single score to represent oral health status. These single scores are, nevertheless, essentially a description of an oral health state, rather than a valuation of it.

Fyffe and Nuttall (1995) have explored the use of valuation techniques in clinical settings, using standard gamble techniques to explore patients' valuations of fillings in comparison to immediate extraction. The context for this work is the use of patients' valuations to help decide which treatment is best for a particular patient. The valuations are specific to treatments, as opposed to oral health states, so do not assist economic evaluation.

Thus, notwithstanding the wide range of generic instruments available to describe oral health QoL, and occasional attempts to explore preferences regarding treatments, the dual elements of description and valuation required in cost utility analysis have not been combined.

This particular gap in the literature has been recognized for some time, and there have been proposals to address it. Kind *et al.* (1998) developed a five-dimension dental health status measure, the DS-QoL, based on the design of the EuroQol EQ-5D. The dimensions are: eating, oral hygiene, aesthetics, pain/discomfort and speech, with three levels in each (no, some and severe problems); in total, 243 oral health states are described. One of these dimensions – oral hygiene – is arguably related to oral health *care* ('I have no/some/I am unable to clean my teeth/mouth') rather than to outcomes as such. Further, the use of the term 'aesthetics' in an instrument intended to be self-completed by the general public is questionable.

A similar but simpler instrument, which may be labelled the Oral Health-3D, comprising just three dimensions and three levels (describing 27 oral health states in total), is proposed in Figure 8.1. Combined with QoL valuation techniques – visual analogue scales, standard gamble or time trade-off – such an approach would be capable of yielding both descriptions and valuations of oral health states for use in economic evaluation. The smaller number of states to be valued simplifies the valuation task; whether this or similar instruments are valid and sufficiently sensitive to changes in oral health states would require testing.

A further, more general problem with measuring and valuing oral health states independently of overall quality of life is that findings cannot facilitate broader assessments of value for money across the health sector, that is the optimal allocation of resources between dental health and other health services remains unidentified. Thus research to develop generic oral health QoL descriptions and valuations should be accompanied by endeavours to establish the correspondence between oral health QoL states and overall QoL measures, such as the EQ-5D, and the valuations assigned to them. More generally, an 'exchange rate' between QALYs and QATYs is required.

An obvious alternative is to eschew generic descriptions and utilities for oral health states (and, by implication, cost utility analysis) and instead seek monetary valuations of oral health improvements. This would overcome the tendency, noted above, for cost–benefit analyses of oral health strategies to rely upon savings as the measure of benefit. Sintonen and Linosmaa (2000) note two reservations about this approach. First, willingness to pay is a function of ability to pay. Second, patients may be less able to value treatments than dentists. Both concerns are common to *all* attempts to elicit the monetary value of health services and outcomes, and are addressed elsewhere in this book (Chapters 1 and 2). However, it is arguable that the lower subsidies that commonly apply to dental care compared to health care generally, and thus patients' experiences of making choices based in part upon the charges which

Oral health questionnaire

We are trying to find out what people think about the state of health of their teeth and gums. We are going to describe some health states that people can be in. We want you to say how good or bad each of these states would be for a person like you. There are no right or wrong answers. We are interested only in your personal view.

But first of all we would like you to indicate below the state of health of your teeth and gums today.

In each of the groups below, please tick the box next to the statement that best describes the health of your teeth and gums today:

Appearance of teeth and gums

I have no problems with the way that my teeth and gums look   ☐

I have some problems with the way that my teeth or gums look   ☐

I have a lot of problems with the way that my teeth or gums look   ☐

Ability to eat and speak

My teeth and gums cause me no problems with eating or speaking   ☐

My teeth or gums cause me some problems with eating or speaking   ☐

My teeth or gums cause me great difficulties in eating or speaking   ☐

Pain and discomfort

I have no pain or discomfort in my teeth and gums   ☐

I have moderate pain or discomfort in my teeth or gums   ☐

I have severe pain or discomfort in my teeth or gums   ☐

Compared with the past 12 months, the general health of my teeth and gums today is

Better   ☐

About the same   ☐

Worse   ☐

Figure 8.1 An example of a generic oral health QoL instrument: the OH-3D

they face, make dental care an obvious candidate for the monetary valuation of benefits.

MEASURING THE PERFORMANCE OF DENTAL HEALTH CARE SYSTEMS

Table 8.1 describes, for OECD countries for which data are available, the total spending on dental care, the contribution of public spending to total dental expenditure, the number of dentists per 1000 population and a measure of oral health of 12-year-olds: the decayed, missing and filled teeth (DMFT) index.

Underlying the variation in the level and sources of spending and the relative abundance of dentists are differences in the mix of ways in which dental care is funded (user charges, social insurance, private insurance and tax-funded subsidization) and provided (by private dentists or other dental workers; practising in private or public clinics) in each country. Such variations are of course evident in health care generally. However, the problems involved in measuring all aspects of health adequately, isolating the effects of health care from other determinants of health and controlling for the effects of ongoing structural reforms to health services all make it difficult to establish cause-and-effect between the characteristics of the system and the efficiency with which it produces health outcomes.

Oral health has an advantage in this context: it is a tightly-defined area of anatomy and service delivery and the measurement of health outcomes is relatively straightforward, with measures being well established and widely used internationally (e.g. DMFT[1]). This makes oral health an ideal 'microcosm' of health services within which to explore methods aimed at linking characteristics of a health care system with health outcomes.

However, simple correlations between the OECD data in Table 8.1 on oral health (DMFT) and dental spending, whether total spending on dental care or the proportion of dental spending which is 'public', fail to reveal any relationship. There are some relationships between other variables: the number of dentists per 10,000 population is significantly negatively correlated with DMFT scores. This might suggest either that supply is following demand, or that dentists cause poor oral health, perhaps through overtreatment. There is a highly significant negative correlation between total spending on dental care per person and the proportion of that spending which is public (excluding Germany, which is an outlier in this regard), although whether this is

---

[1] Although DMFT (decayed, missing and filled teeth) is a widely accepted and commonly used measure of oral health, there are some problems with relying on this as a measure of oral health. These are discussed in the first section of this chapter.

Table 8.1 Indicators of dental care inputs and oral health outcomes

Country	Total spending on dental care per capita, US$ (purchasing power parity)	Public spending as a % total dental care spending	Spending on dental care as a % all health care spending	Dentists per 1000 population	Oral health (average DMFT at age 12)
Australia	$102 [98]	13.9% [98]	4.9% [98]	0.4 [97]	0.9 [97]
Austria	n.a	n.a	n.a	**0.5**	1.7 [97]
Canada	**$186**	**5.6%**	**7.6%**	0.5 [98]	n.a
Czech Republic	**$53**	**57.1%**	**5.4%**	**0.6**	3.2 [97]
Denmark	n.a	n.a	n.a	0.9 [98]	**1.0**
Finland	**$95**	**34.2%**	**6.1%**	**0.9**	1.1 [97]
France	**$107**	34.3% [97]	**5.0%**	0.7 [97]	2.1 [93]
Germany	$250 [98]	55.1% [98]	10.6% [98]	0.8 [98]	1.7 [97]
Greece	$35 [92]	n.a	n.a	1.1 [97]	1.6 [93]
Hungary	n.a	n.a	n.a	**0.5**	3.7 [96]
Iceland	**$175**	**21.7%**	**7.7%**	1.0 [98]	1.5 [96]
Ireland	$44 [92]	31.3% [92]	4.1% [92]	**0.5**	1.8 [92]
Italy	n.a	n.a	n.a	**0.6**	2.1 [96]
Japan	$121 [98]	78.3% [98]	6.7% [98]	0.7 [98]	**2.4**
Luxembourg	**$62**	**84.8%**	**2.4%**	**0.6**	**0.7**
Netherlands	**$85**	**28.2%**	**3.8%**	**0.5**	**1.0**
New Zealand	n.a	n.a	n.a	**0.4**	1.6 [97]
Norway	$54 [91]	67.3% [88]	n.a	n.a	1.6 [98]
Poland	n.a.	n.a	n.a	**0.3**	5.1 [91]
Portugal	n.a	n.a	n.a	0.3 [98]	3.2 [90]
Spain	n.a	n.a	n.a	0.4 [98]	2.3 [94]
Sweden	$148 [92]	n.a	9.8% [92]	0.9 [98]	**0.9**
Switzerland	$237 [98]	7.3% [98]	8.3% [98]	0.5 [98]	n.a
Turkey	n.a	n.a	n.a	**0.2**	2.7 [90]
United Kingdom	$63 [92]	48.4% [92]	5.4% [92]	**0.4**	1.1 [96]
United States	**$206**	**4.6%**	**4.7%**	0.6 [98]	n.a

Note: Figures in bold are for 1999 (the most recent year for which a reasonable number of observations are available on dental care spending). In other cases, the most recent figure is provided and the period to which it corresponds shown in brackets – comparisons should therefore be approached with caution.
Source: OECD 2001 Health Data.

attributable to public systems being more efficient or facing tighter budget constraints remains speculative.

The difficulty in identifying and explaining complex relationships between oral health and 'system' variables in such a manner suggests a more systematic approach to explaining variations in oral health is required. The literature on international comparisons of health system efficiency (for example, WHO 2000; Feachem *et al.* 2002) is mostly inconclusive not only because of deficiencies in data, but also because of the lack of an adequate analytical framework (Parkin 1989). The RAND Health Insurance Experiment (Newhouse 1993) provides evidence on the links between alternative insurance

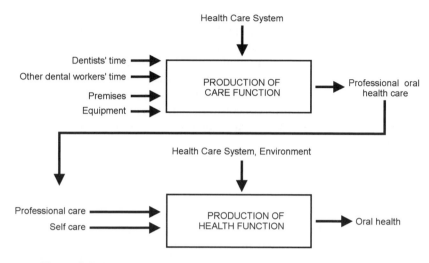

Figure 8.2 A model of the production of oral health and dental health care

arrangements, demand and health – but provides limited insights into the performance of alternative 'whole systems' for funding and delivering care, and on the effects of wider environmental factors.

To address this, a model is proposed comprising two linked production processes: the production of dental health care and of dental health. The model builds upon existing work on the demand for health (Grossman 1972) and on health determinants (Evans & Stoddart 1990). Figure 8.2 illustrates the model.

The model recognizes that, in explaining the relationship between oral health and the oral health care system, there are two production processes of concern: the production of oral health *care*, and the production of oral *health*. Professional health care is created by the formal health care system, using inputs such as dentists' and other oral health workers' time, equipment, premises and consumables. Oral health is created by individuals who utilize the output of oral health care and combine this with inputs supplied by themselves – for example, personal oral hygiene.

The two processes are linked, by recognizing that the output of the oral health care production function is an input to the oral health production function. The variables of most interest are key features of the oral health care system that, along with broadly defined environmental factors such as those covered in depth by the health determinants literature, affect both processes as mediating factors. In effect, there are two submodels, which together form an overall system.

The model suggests the variables of interest in empirical work (including key features of the oral health care system which, along with socio-economic influences and other health determinants affect both submodels) and provides a conceptual basis for empirically testable hypotheses concerning the effect of health system characteristics on oral health.

In the following sections two original applications of the model are reported, each employing different approaches to empirical testing. The data were collected on a pilot basis only and are not appropriate for sophisticated analysis and for drawing firm conclusions. The intention is to demonstrate directions and challenges facing research on this topic; results should be viewed as illustrative only.

DATA

Data from France, Denmark, Germany, Ireland, Netherlands, Spain and the United Kingdom were collected in 1994 as part of a EU BIOMED project (EOHC 1997). These data facilitated the construction of relevant variables for dental practices, the health care production model, households (for the health production model) and the country level for system features. The data had a multilevel structure, comprising seven countries, 287 dental practices and 1392 patients. Some, though not all, of the data could be linked between patients and their dentists and vice versa. It should be noted that the data were not collected using fully random procedures, and are therefore not to be taken as representative. Details of the samples available for analysis are presented in Table 8.2.

There are several limitations of this data set. First, only patients and dentists within the social security scheme of each country were included. The key characteristics of these, as they were at the time that the data were collected,

Table 8.2 Numbers included in a sample of dentists and patients in seven European Union countries

Country	Dentists			Patients		
	Total	No missing data	Linked to patients	Total	No missing data	
Denmark	51	27	0	85	72	
France	45	35	29	303	201	
Germany	46	42	12	273	231	
Ireland	42	38	19	307	228	
Netherlands	46	44	9	279	227	
Spain	57	57	18	241	199	
UK	51	44	19	274	234	
TOTAL	338	287	108	1762	1392	

Box 8.2 Key features of the funding and provision of oral health services in European countries in 1994

France: A social security system, based on private care with a mandatory insurance system covering the population and financed by taxes. A small number are entitled to free care but fixed tooth replacements and prosthesis are paid for by patients, the majority of whom have private insurance. For all other activities patients pay all fees to the dentist, who may choose the level of fees, then have 75% reimbursed by the social security system.

Denmark: A national health insurance scheme, which operates a system of co-payments for oral care. Dentists are paid on a fee per item basis.

Germany: A sick fund insurance system, which 90% of citizens are members of. Most services are covered by the sick funds, with a 50% contribution for prosthetic services.

Ireland: A social welfare dental benefit scheme, using a system of co-payments with patients paying on average one-third of costs. Dentists are paid on an agreed scheme of fees per item.

The Netherlands: A national health insurance scheme, covering 62% of the population, the majority of the rest having private insurance. Dentists are reimbursed on a fee schedule for those covered by the scheme and by direct payment for those not covered (this system has since changed and most adults now have private insurance to cover most treatments).

Spain: A social security system, covering the entire population with salaried dentists.

UK: A National Health Service covering over 70% of registered dentists who receive over 90% of remuneration on a fees per item basis. 66% of fees come from tax-based public funding and 34% through patient fees. 79% of patients pay full charges for services, the rest are either fully or partly covered.

are described in Box 8.2. Second, a key environmental factor – fluoridation of water supplies – is unable to be included as there is insufficient variation between the sample countries. Similarly, other important system characteristics – such as the effects of regulations restricting entry to the dental profession – could not be included. Third, the data provide a 'snap shot' of factors hypothesized to influence oral health, whereas oral health will be a function of both current and lagged determinants, including previous oral health.

APPLICATION 1: REGRESSION MODELLING

An obvious approach is to choose a single dependent variable and use regression techniques to investigate the influence of each independent variable suggested by the conceptual model in Figure 8.2. The production of oral health care is based on the dental practice; the production of oral health is based on the household. In both cases mediating factors operate at the national level, describing the oral health care system and other environmental factors. Estimation of the model's parameters gives rise to a large number of technical and statistical problems. These include aggregation, simultaneous equations, multiple outcome indicators and the modelling strategy to be adopted.

The aggregation issue concerns the fact that the submodels are at different levels of aggregation, and the system and some environmental variables are at yet another level of aggregation. A simple solution to this, which would enable system characteristics to be related to outcomes, is to regard system characteristics as fixed effects that alter the relationship between health inputs and health outputs. This is illustrated in Figure 8.3. A better statistical solution would be to employ multilevel modelling; unfortunately, the sample size and other characteristics of these pilot study data do not permit sophisticated analyses of that kind.

Figure 8.3 suggests a positive relationship between health inputs and outputs in two different oral health care systems, but that system 1 produces more outputs per unit of input than system 2. A regression approach should enable this difference to be quantified. However, the fact that the system variables in practice essentially relate to countries means that in effect the modelling may reduce to an international comparison of systems, which could obscure the different effects of different system features.

The approach outlined suggests estimation of two models, which together form a system. The alternative of having one model (a 'reduced form') might be easier, but would suffer from problems of interpretability. It is therefore necessary to estimate the structural equations deriving from the two models, the deterministic elements of which are:

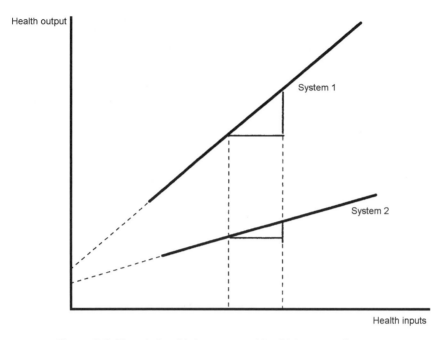

Figure 8.3 The relationship between oral health inputs and outputs

$$\text{Care} = \alpha + \beta * X \qquad (8.1)$$

$$\text{Health} = \gamma + \delta * \text{Care} + \varepsilon * Y \qquad (8.2)$$

where Care is a variable representing the amount of oral health care produced, X is a vector describing the factors influencing care, Health is a variable representing the amount of oral health produced, Y is a vector describing factors other than oral health care which influence health, and α, β, γ, δ and ε are the estimated parameters of the model.

In order to avoid the mismatch between the level of aggregation of dental practices and households, a possible alternative would be to estimate the structural equations separately. However, this would give incorrect estimates. A solution to this is to employ two-stage least squares. Unfortunately, the necessity then to employ multilevel modelling makes the estimation process far more complex. In either case, the data simply do not permit such analyses.

The problem of multiple outcome indicators arises because a single or encompassing measure of oral health is not available. As a result, a number of models are required to be estimated. This extensive use of the data set increases the problem of interpreting results, because repeatedly testing a single set of hypotheses using the same data increases the possibility of a Type 2 error.

Finally, there is the issue of which modelling strategy is to be adopted. This in itself involves a number of issues that affect the actual form of the model that is to be estimated and used as the set of results. It includes which variables are to be included in the equations and the functional form of the equations. The general approach adopted here (subject to the warning given earlier that the actual modelling is exploratory and illustrative) is a rudimentary general-to-specific approach relying on diagnostic testing of the validity of the model to assess its validity.

As a result of the data limitations, the most simple of regression procedures were employed, to illustrate the potential of the approach. Variables used in the estimation of equations (8.1) and (8.2) are defined in Tables 8.3 and 8.4.

RESULTS

Results from the estimation of equations (8.1) and (8.2) are shown in Tables 8.5–8.7.[2]

Table 8.5 shows the results from OLS regression carried out using the measure of oral health care (OUTPUT). The parameter estimates (coefficients) are given, along with their standard errors; a t-test is used to test for significance. Equation diagnostics are given in terms of the goodness of fit (R^2, adjusted R^2, F-test).

Two different estimates are given. The first includes all of the variables except the system variables and the second includes all of the variables except the country variables. There are few differences in the parameter estimates of those variables included in both equations or in the test diagnostics. However, from the point of view of our aims, the second is much more informative.

Consistent findings from the country and system models are that the amount of time spent by dentists chairside and in administration have a negative effect on the production of health care, suggesting these inputs may experience diminishing marginal products. The country model suggests that French dental care is more productive and Irish and Dutch less productive – however, this in itself is not very informative without knowing the characteristics of the dental care systems in each case. For the system model, all of the coefficients are significant. These suggest the lower the ratio of population to dentists, the higher the average age of dentists, the more preventively oriented the fee structure and the lower the patient contribution to treatment costs, the greater the output of the system. These results provide much more insight into the determinants of system productivity.

[2] Results from alternative specifications of all regressions (for example, excluding the country variables, and estimates for significant variables only, following stepwise regression) are not reported here, but are broadly consistent with the results in Tables 8.5–8.8.

Table 8.3 Dependent and independent variables for the production of oral health care model

Dependent variable:	
OUTPUT	Average number of patients seen per hour worked in system by each dentist

Independent variables:	
DENT_AGE	Average age of dentists in system
EQUIP_AGE	Age of dental unit
HRS_CHAIR	Average number of hours per week worked by dentists chairside
HRS_ADMIN	Average number of hours per week worked by dentists administration, etc.
CHAIRS	Number of chairs concurrently operated by dentist
STAFFHOURSa– STAFFHOURSe	Time worked by various support staff: a = reception staff b = chairside assistants c = hygienists d = staff conducting health education e = 'other tasks'
STAFFHOURS	Total time worked by support staff: sum of STAFFHOURSa– STAFFHOURSe
WEEKSWORKED	Average number of weeks worked per year by each dentist
YEARSEXP	Number of years spent practising since qualifying by each dentist
POPRATIO	Population per dentist in system
PYINDEX	System denture fee as multiple of filling fee
COPAYMENT	Whether or not patients contribute to treatment cost

Table 8.4 Dependent and independent variables for the production of oral health model

Dependent variables:	
STATE	State of teeth and gums, 1 = excellent or good for both, 0 = average or poor for teeth or gums or both
SOUND	Number of sound unrestored teeth

Independent variables:	
AGE	1 = 35–44, 0 = 20–24
ATTEND	Visited dental practice, 1 = Yes, 0 = No
BRUSH	Brush teeth, 1 = once a day or more, 0 = less often
CHECK	Check up last two years, 1 = Yes, 0 = No
CONSND	Consulted non-dentist, 1 = Yes, 0 = No
EDUC	1 = Third level, etc., 0 = primary or secondary
EMPLOY	1 = Fixed employment, 0 = occasional employment or unemployed
SATIS	1 = Satisfied or very satisfied for all aspects of service, 0 = dissatisfied or very dissatisfied for at least one aspect
SEX	1 = Female, 0 = Male
FEES	% Expenditure borne by patient fees
PYINDEX	System denture fee as multiple of filling fee
SUGARPC	Sugar consumption in country, kg per person

Table 8.5 OLS regression analyses for production of health care model

Variable	Country model		System model	
CHAIRS	−0.014	(0.123)	0.029	(0.119)
EQUIP_AGE	0.049	(0.049)	0.049	(0.049)
YEARSEXP	−0.016	(0.035)	−0.013	(0.034)
HRS_CHAIR	**−0.280**	**(0.030)**	**−0.294**	**(0.028)**
HRS_ADMIN	**−0.187**	**(0.057)**	**−0.205**	**(0.056)**
STAFFHOURSa	0.026	(0.022)	0.028	(0.021)
STAFFHOURSb	0.001	(0.018)	−0.003	(0.018)
STAFFHOURSc	0.032	(0.040)	0.036	(0.040)
STAFFHOURSd	0.001	(0.056)	−0.010	(0.056)
STAFFHOURSe	0.059	(0.034)	0.054	(0.034)
WEEKSWORKED	0.118	(0.073)	0.125	(0.073)
DENMARK	−0.736	(1.218)		
FRANCE	**7.526**	**(1.177)**		
GERMANY	1.035	(1.034)		
IRELAND	**−4.839**	**(1.168)**		
NETHERLANDS	*−2.498*	*(1.084)*		
SPAIN	−0.371	(1.214)		
POPRATIO			**−0.007**	**(0.001)**
DENT_AGE			**0.709**	**(0.161)**
PYINDEX			**−0.154**	**(0.025)**
COPAYMENT			**−0.176**	**(0.020)**
Constant	5.929	(3.539)	−0.376	9.486
Observations	316			
R-squared	**0.526**		**0.522**	
Adjusted *R*-squared	**0.499**		**0.498**	
F-statistic	**19.43**		**21.83**	

Standard errors in parentheses.
Bold: significant at $p < 0.01$.
Bold and italic: significant at $p < 0.05$.

Table 8.6 shows the results from a logistic regression carried out using the patient-based measure of oral health (STATE). Because this is a binary variable the estimate is of the probability of having a good state of oral health. The coefficients, expressed as the logarithm of the odds of having good oral health, and their standard errors are given; a Wald test is used to test significance. Equation diagnostics are given in terms of goodness of fit χ^2 and the percentage of correct classifications by the model to the dichotomous dependent variable.

The results concerning countries are consistent with the production of oral health care model: France is more productive, and the Netherlands, along with Spain, less productive. The system variables are of potential interest, but only one is significant: higher sugar consumption leads to worse oral health. Consistent findings between the models are that older people and those who

Table 8.6 Logistic regression analyses for production of health model

Variable	Country model		System model	
AGE	−0.652	(0.113)	−0.642	(0.112)
ATTEND	0.129	(0.312)	0.234	(0.311)
BRUSH	0.010	(0.201)	**0.438**	**(0.160)**
CHECK	0.375	(0.212)	0.389	(0.212)
CONSND	−0.534	(0.255)	−0.502	(0.254)
EDUC	−0.053	(0.122)	−0.154	(0.118)
EMPLOY	0.284	(0.123)	0.257	(0.122)
SATIS	0.147	(0.126)	0.113	(0.124)
SEX	0.136	(0.114)	0.096	(0.113)
DENMARK	0.327	(0.312)		
FRANCE	−0.488	(0.246)		
GERMANY	−0.475	(0.246)		
IRELAND	0.356	(0.232)		
NETHERLANDS	**0.709**	**(0.249)**		
SPAIN	**0.751**	**(0.251)**		
FEES			−0.857	(0.534)
PYINDEX			−0.004	(0.003)
SUGARPC			**0.145**	**(0.026)**
Constant	0.071	(0.402)	−5.36	**(0.916)**
Observations	1501		1501	
Log likelihood	−963.36		−976.30	
Goodness of fit χ^2	450.90		485.00	
Correctly classified	62.82%		62.76%	

Standard errors in parentheses.
Bold: significant at $p < 0.01$.
Bold and italic: significant at $p < 0.05$.

have consulted a non-dentist have worse oral health, and those who are in fixed employment have better oral health. A further finding from the system model is that those who brush their teeth more often have better oral health.

Finally, Table 8.7 shows the results from OLS regression carried out using the dentist-based measure of oral health (SOUND). Results concerning countries are consistent in the direction of effect with the previous model, although a different pattern of significance emerges. Within the system model, the preventive orientation of the system emerges as the only significant variable, consistent with the production of health care model. Again, higher age and consultation with a non-dentist led to lower dental health, while women have worse oral health than men. For the country model only, attendance at dental practices appears to be associated with worse oral health and higher education with better oral health.

This description of the analyses which were feasible given the data set demonstrates the huge problems which would be faced in obtaining more

Table 8.7 OLS regression analyses for production of health model

Variable	Country model		System model	
AGE	−7.34	(0.317)	−7.376	(0.322)
ATTEND	−2.01	(0.832)	−1.331	(0.840)
BRUSH	0.207	(0.562)	0.448	(0.456)
CHECK	−0.026	(0.581)	0.015	(0.592)
CONSND	−2.176	(0.687)	−2.174	(0.700)
EDUC	1.129	(0.348)	0.627	(0.345)
EMPLOY	−0.230	(0.349)	−0.430	(0.354)
SATIS	−0.408	(0.354)	−0.630	(0.360)
SEX	−1.242	(0.322)	−1.32	(0.327)
DENMARK	1.850	(0.897)		
FRANCE	−1.428	(0.702)		
GERMANY	−2.656	(0.706)		
IRELAND	0.069	(0.664)		
NETHERLANDS	0.584	(0.702)		
SPAIN	4.296	(0.699)		
FEES			−1.688	(1.571)
PYINDEX			−0.075	(0.010)
SUGARPC			−0.080	(0.074)
Constant	31.76	(1.11)	37.22	(2.58)
Observations	1489			
R-squared	0.352		0.325	
Adjusted R-squared	0.345		0.320	
F-statistic	53.22		59.27	

Standard errors in parentheses.
Bold: significant at $p < 0.01$.
Bold and italic: significant at $p < 0.05$.

trustworthy estimates. Data requirements would be onerous, both in terms of sample sizes required and in terms of management to ensure coordination and consistency between different levels. Although many of the individual data items require close attention to definitional problems, this is particularly acute for outcome measures. However, there is an additional crucial dimension, which has not been dealt with at all here: people's oral health is the result of the history of their actions and interactions with the environment and health system. Introducing time and an associated life-cycle model multiplies the complexity and empirical difficulties.

APPLICATION 2: DATA ENVELOPMENT ANALYSIS

Various methods exist to explore efficiency other than standard regression production function models, including stochastic frontiers and data envelopment analysis (DEA). Each has been used to explore the production of dental care (Buck 2000; Grytten 2000; Grytten & Rongen 2000; Sintonen & Linosmaa 2000). In this application DEA is used to explore the relative efficiency of different oral health *systems*. The principal advantage of DEA is its ability to deal with multiple outputs. This method has been described in detail elsewhere (Parkin & Hollingsworth 1997); a brief description follows.

DEA is a non-parametric technique that uses linear programming to construct an efficiency frontier based on best practice. For a multiple-output, multiple-input firm such as a dental practice, which treats different sorts of conditions using different staff, equipment and materials, a measure of technical efficiency (TE) is:

$$\text{TE} = \frac{\sum\limits_{r=1}^{p} y_r}{\sum\limits_{i=1}^{m} x_i} \qquad (8.3)$$

where i indexes inputs x and r indexes outputs y. Heterogeneous inputs and outputs cannot be simply summed, so weights are assigned to each input and output such that:

$$\text{TE} = \frac{\sum\limits_{r=1}^{p} u_r y_r}{\sum\limits_{i=1}^{m} v_i x_i} \qquad (8.4)$$

where y_r is output r, u_r is the weight attached to output r, x_i is input i, v_i is the weight attached to input i, and where the weights are specific to each firm, or unit. DEA estimates this measure of technical efficiency for each unit. A higher value means greater efficiency and it is bounded by 0 and 100%, the latter indicating full efficiency.

In this application DEA is used to examine the efficiency with which different systems produce oral health care and oral health. The variables used to measure this were those found to be significant in the above regression analyses.

The *input* variables for the production of care model were CHAIRS, DENT_AGE, YEARSEXP and the total of STAFFHOURSa to STAFF-HOURSe. The output measure was OUTPUT. For the subsample of dentists whose data could be linked to patient data (see Table 8.2), indicators of the quality of their patients' oral health were included. These were aggregated from the variables SOUND and STATE.

The input variables for the production of health model were BRUSH, CHECK, CONSND and EMPLOY. Output variables were SOUND and

STATE. The latter is a categorical variable, to which the normal DEA procedure cannot be applied. A two-stage DEA procedure was therefore devised. First, a DEA frontier was estimated for the subsample of those assessed to be in a poor state. This ensures that the efficiency scores are relative to those with a similar poor state of health. Second, the whole sample were analysed together. The efficiency scores of those with good oral health were taken from this analysis.

It is possible to estimate these models within countries and this is valuable for some purposes. However, such models cannot be compared *between* countries because the different best-practice production frontiers have no common base. Therefore both the oral health care and oral health production models were estimated using pooled data to form a single cross-country production function. Spain's system is largely an extraction-only service, in contrast to the comprehensive dental services provided in the other countries. Efficiency comparisons with respect to the production of health care are therefore confounded by the fact that the output in Spain is much less complex. The same applies to the production of health, not because the inputs or outputs differ from other countries, but because the *mix* of cases seen within the system is different. Therefore, although calculations were carried out on the whole data set, results presented here exclude Spain. As there were no linked data from Denmark, it is excluded from the quality adjusted health care production model.

RESULTS

Table 8.8 shows the median efficiency scores and the number of practices efficient within the different countries. For the production of health care, the UK has the highest average score and UK dentists form a large majority of the best practice frontier. Germany has the lowest average score, and has no practices on the best practice frontier.

The results when this model was estimated *including* data from Spain are as expected. Spain had the highest median efficiency score (24.8), although not much higher than that of the UK (20.5). This reflects the relative ease of obtaining output for a given set of inputs, manifested as apparently highly efficient units. All the median scores were much lower (for the whole sample, 14.8 compared with 37.6) reflecting the existence of those same units. However, the ranking of other countries was not affected, suggesting that the analysis for them was not affected by the inclusion of irrelevant alternatives.

The absolute values of efficiency for the quality adjusted health care model cannot be compared with the previous model because of the smaller numbers of practices included. The rankings are, however, identical, and France now supplies the largest number of practices on the efficiency frontier. Germany

Table 8.8 Comparative efficiency of six European Union countries in the production of oral health care, quality adjusted oral health care and oral health

	Oral health care				Quality adjusted oral health care				Oral health		
	N	Median score	Number efficient		N	Median score	Number efficient		N	Median score	Number efficient
UK	44	67.93	14	UK	19	100	13	UK	234	53.33	10
Ireland	38	48.53	3	Ireland	19	93.61	5	Denmark	72	53.21	1
Nether-lands	44	40.22	1	Nether-lands	9	84.48	3	Ireland	228	50.00	6
France	35	35.36	3	France	29	75.00	5	Nether-lands	227	50.00	2
Denmark	27	29.79	1	Germany	12	44.52	0	France	201	43.75	4
Germany	42	24.08	0					Germany	231	41.94	3
All	230	38.62	22	All	88	84.88	26	All	1193	48.31	26

retains its low average score and lack of efficient practices. As explained above, this model excludes Denmark. To enable a proper comparison, the non-quality adjusted models were re-estimated without Denmark; this had no impact on the countries' rankings.

There is relatively little variation in efficiency between countries in the production of oral health, but the UK again has the highest average score and France and Germany have the lowest. UK patients also supply the largest number of those on the health production efficiency frontier, but otherwise the numbers who are efficient in each country again do not follow the efficiency score rankings. Again, when Spain was included it had the highest average score and the most efficient practices, but other countries' rankings were unaltered.

As with the regression analyses, the results should be treated with caution because of the size and non-random nature of the samples on which they are based. They do, however, illustrate the potential value of the approach. They suggest a reasonable correlation between the efficiency with which dentists in a country produce oral health care and the efficiency with which their patients produce oral health.

While the results from Applications 1 and 2 are tentative, they demonstrate the potential insights into the influence of health systems on health outcomes that are possible. Identification of the dental practice, household and system variables that exert the greatest effect on oral health can inform policy aimed at improving oral health. However, whether modifying these variables is efficient depends on what specific interventions exist and their relative effectiveness and cost. Economic evaluation is required to address these questions.

164   ADVANCES IN HEALTH ECONOMICS

CONCLUSION

Production function approaches grounded in theory provide a way of systematically exploring the effects of, and interactions between, household, dental practice and system-wide factors on oral health. These can be used to identify the variables that exert the greatest influence on oral health.

Which strategies are efficient to pursue in modifying these variables depends on their relative cost and effectiveness. Existing approaches to the measurement and valuation of oral health outcomes limit the ability of economic evaluation to inform oral health policy and to determine the appropriate allocation of scarce health resources between oral health and other health care services. An important area for future research is the development of valuations for oral health states. This could proceed by eliciting utilities for generically described oral health QoL, and the establishment of 'exchange rates' between these and generic health-related QoL valuations. Alternatively, patients' willingness to pay for improvements in oral health could be sought. Either approach would serve to improve the quality of economic evaluations and to inform the allocation of resources to and between oral health care programmes.

ACKNOWLEDGEMENTS

The second section of this chapter is based upon an original paper jointly written by the authors and Bruce Hollingsworth. We are grateful to Bruce for allowing its inclusion here. The EU BIOMED programme provided initial funding for this project to the consortium 'Efficiency in Oral Health Care. The Evaluation of Oral Health Systems in Europe', who collected the data and contributed to development of the theoretical model. We acknowledge and thank members of the consortium, particularly Professor Denis O'Mullane, Dr Helen Whelton, Professor Martin Downer and Mr Mark Deverill. We are grateful to John Forbes and the editors for helpful comments on an earlier draft of this chapter.

REFERENCES

Adulyanon S, Vourapukjaru J and Sheiham A (1996) Oral impacts affecting daily performance in a low dental disease Thai population. *Community Dentistry and Oral Epidemiology*, **24**, 385–389.
Antczak-Bouckoms AA and Weinstein MC (1987) Cost effectiveness analysis of periodontal disease control. *Journal of Dental Research*, **66**, 1630–1635.
Arinen SS and Sintonen H (1995) *Does the 15D register variation in oral health?* Abstract Book ISTAHC 11th annual meeting, Stockholm, Sweden, June 4–7, p. 155.

Atchison A and Dolan TA (1990) Development of the Geriatric Oral Health Assessment Index. *Journal of Dental Education*, **54**, 680–687.

Birch S (1986) Measuring dental health: improvements on the DMF index. *Community Dental Health*, **3**, 303–311.

Buck D (2000) The efficiency of the community dental service in England: a data envelopment analysis. *Community Dentistry and Oral Epidemiology*, **28**(4), 274–280.

Cooper MH (1980) The demand and need for dental care. In RAB Leaper (Ed.), *Health, Wealth and Housing*. Blackwell, Oxford.

Cushing A, Sheiham A and Maizels J (1986) Developing socio-dental indicators – the social impact of dental disease. *Community Dental Health*, **3**, 3–17.

Davis P (1981) Culture, inequality and the pattern of dental care in New Zealand. *Social Science and Medicine*, **15**, 801–805.

Devlin N, Parkin D and Yule B (2002) *The Economics of Oral Health and Dental Care*. University of Otago Press, Dunedin, New Zealand.

EOHC (Efficiency in Oral Health Care Project) (1997) *The evaluation of oral health systems in Europe*. EU BIOMED project report, Dental Health Services Research Unit, University College Cork.

Evans R and Stoddart G (1990) Producing health, consuming health care. *Social Science and Medicine*, **31**(12), 1347–1363.

Feacham RGA, Sehri NK and White KL (2002) Getting more for their dollar: a comparison of the NHS with California's Kaiser Permanante. *British Medical Journal*, **324**, 135–143.

Fyffe, HE and Nuttall NM (1995) Decision processes in the management of dental disease. Part 1: QALYs, QATYs and dental health state utilities. *Dental Update*, **22**(2), 67–71.

Gray AM (1982) The production of dental care in the British NHS. *Scottish Journal of Political Economy*, **29**, 59–74.

Grossman M (1972) On the concept of health capital and the demand for health. *Journal of Political Economy*, **80**, 223–255.

Grytten J (2000) Production frontier analyses: comments on the methodology. *Community Dentistry and Oral Epidemiology*, **28**(2), 81–82.

Grytten J and Rongen G (2000) Efficiency in the provision of public dental services in Norway. *Community Dentistry and Oral Epidemiology*, **28**(3), 170–176.

Kind P, Boyd T and Corson M (1998) Measuring dental health status: calibrating a context-specific instrument. In W Greiner, J-M Graf v.d. Schulenburg and J Piercy (Eds), *Proceedings of the 15th Scientific Plenary of the EuroQol Group*. University of Hanover, Hanover.

Leao A and Sheiham A (1996) The development of a socio-dental measure of dental impacts on daily living. *Community Dental Health*, **13**(1), 22–26.

Locker D (1995) Health outcomes of oral disorders. *International Journal of Epidemiology*, **24**(3), S85–S89.

McGrath C and Bedi R (2001) An evaluation of a new measure of oral health related quality of life – OHQoL – UK(W). *Community Dental Health*, **18**(3), 138–143.

Newhouse JP (1993) *Free for All? Lessons from RAND Health Insurance Experiment*. Harvard University Press, Cambridge, MA.

Parkin D (1989) Comparing health service efficiency across countries. *Oxford Review of Economic Policy*, **5**(1), 75–88.

Parkin D and Hollingsworth B (1997) Measuring production efficiency of acute hospitals in Scotland, 1991–94: validity issues in data envelopment analysis. *Applied Economics*, **29**, 1425–1433.

Parkin D and Yule B (1986) *Financing of Dental Care in Europe: Part 1*. World Health Organisation, Copenhagen.

Parkin D and Yule B (1988) Patient charges and the demand for dental care in Scotland 1962–1981. *Applied Economics*, **20**, 229–242.

Reisine S and Weber J (1989) The impact of dental conditions on patients' quality of life. *Community Dental and Oral Epidemiology*, **17**, 7–10.

Rosenberg D, Kaplan S, Senie R and Badner V (1988) Relationships among dental functional status, clinical dental measures and generic health measures. *Journal of Dental Education*, **11**, 653–657.

Sintonen H and Linosmaa I (2000) Economics of dental services. In AJ Culyer and JP Newhouse (Eds), *Handbook of Health Economics, Volume 1b*. North-Holland, Amsterdam.

Slade GD (1997) Derivation and validation of a short-form Oral Health Impact Profile. *Community Dentistry and Oral Epidemiology*, **25**(4), 284–290.

Slade GD and Spencer AJ (1994) Development and evaluation of the Oral Health Impact Profile. *Community Health Dentistry*, **11**, 3–11.

Spolsky VW, Konberg KJ and Lohr KN (1983) *Measurement of Dental Health Status*. Rand, Santa Monica.

WHO (2000) *Health Systems: Improving Performance*. WHO, Geneva.

Yule B (1984) Need and decision making in dentistry – an economics perspective. *International Dental Journal*, **34**(3), 219–223.

Yule B (1988) *Financing of Dental Care in Europe: Part 2*. World Health Organisation, Copenhagen.

Yule BF and Parkin D (1985) The demand for dental care: an assessment. *Social Science and Medicine*, **21**(7), 753–760.

Yule BF, van Amerongen BM and van Schaik MC (1986) The economics and evaluation of dental care and treatment. *Social Science and Medicine* **22**(11), 1131–1139.

Yule BF, Ryan ME and Parkin DW (1988) Patient charges and the use of dental services: some evidence. *British Dental Journal*, **165**(10), 376–379.

9

Ageing, Disability and Long-term Care Expenditures

PAUL McNAMEE

Health Economics Research Unit, University of Aberdeen

SALLY C. STEARNS

Department of Health Policy and Administration, University of North Carolina at Chapel Hill

INTRODUCTION

Several demographic trends in developed countries are expected to exert greater pressures on the financing and delivery of formal care services for older people. First, the post-war baby boom generation is approaching retirement, so the absolute number of older people will continue to rise. Second, mortality rates have fallen over time. In particular, declines in mortality over the last 40 years have been increasingly accounted for by mortality declines among older people (Cutler & Meara 2001), adding further to the older population. Finally, fertility rates have been in steady decline over the past three decades. Since health and long-term care use increases with age, these trends may culminate in an increasingly disproportionate aggregate demand for services by older retired people relative to the working population available to finance the additional services.

This chapter reviews the literature in order to examine critically (1) the assumptions and methods used in studies that measure the projected demographic trends and (2) the implications of such trends for health and social care expenditures for older people.

Table 9.1 shows how these trends have led to increasing numbers of older people as a proportion of the overall population, particularly within the UK. With 15.7% of the population over age 65 in 1996, the UK is already an 'old' country relative to the US. The proportion of the population that is above the

Advances in Health Economics. Edited by Anthony Scott, Alan Maynard and Robert Elliott.
© 2003 John Wiley & Sons, Ltd

Table 9.1 Population and age structure of countries in the OECD, 1996

Country	Population (thousands)	Age structure of population (% of total population)		
		Under 15	15–64	65 and over
United Kingdom	58,782	19.3	64.9	15.7
United States	265,557	21.7	65.5	12.8
G7	677,897	18.9	66.9	14.2
EU-15	373,220	17.4	67.1	15.5
OECD Total	1,092,208	21.5	66.9	12.6

Source: Reproduced from Rosenberg (2000).
Original Source: Labour Force Statistics, 1976–1996; OECD, Paris, 1997.

state retirement age in the UK is also higher than the average among the 15 European Union countries, for which 15.5% of the population was aged 65 and over.

The World Bank (1999) also provides estimates of the proportion of the population aged 65 years or over among the seven richest industrialized 'G7' countries. These data, summarized in Figure 9.1 for 2000, 2020 and 2040, show that the UK can expect to see the share of the older population grow, but that the proportion of the older population by 2040 is expected to be lower than other G7 nations, except for the US.

Other socio-economic changes are also likely to have an impact on the demand for formal care. The proportion of people living alone has been increasing (Evandrou & Falkingham 2000), and there may be fewer people able to supply informal care, particularly as non-elderly females increase their labour force participation (OECD 1996).

COSTS AND THE DEMOGRAPHIC 'TIME BOMB'

These developments are usually taken to imply that there will be greater problems for the financing and delivery of health and social services in future years. A demographic 'time bomb' is often assumed to be ticking away (McLoughlin 1991; Raleigh 1997). These problems emerge from an extrapolation of current estimates of age-based expenditures per capita or the proportion of expenditures accounted for by older age groups relative to the proportion of older people in the population. Between 1996 and 1999, the average annual cost to the National Health Service (NHS) among persons aged 85 years or over was around £2100 per capita, which was four times the cost for those aged 45–64 years and six times higher than those 16–44 years (Wanless 2002). In addition, although approximately one-fifth of the UK population is

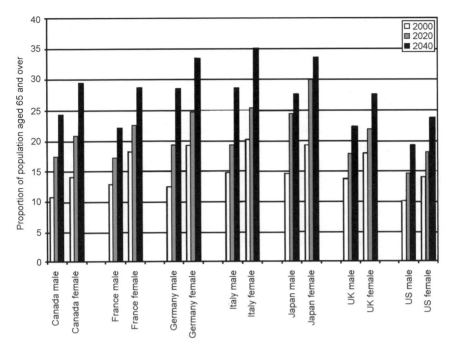

Figure 9.1 Predicted growth in proportion of population aged 65 and over, G7 countries
Source: World Bank (1999). Projections use a net reproduction rate = 1 by 2035

aged 65 years or over, this group accounted for around 40% of hospital and community health services and almost 50% of social services expenditure in 1998–1999 (Department of Health 2001). The Organisation for Economic Cooperation and Development (OECD) estimates that although EU countries currently spend less than 2% of GDP on long-term care (OECD 1998a, p. 98), these costs will increase by 50% over the next 20 to 30 years. Even so, future long-term care spending may remain below 2% of GDP in most countries.

POLICY RESPONSES

Empirical data such as these have, in part, led policy-makers at the national level to enact recent legislative changes relating to taxation, pension policy and methods of health and social care organization (OECD 1996, 2000). In the UK, these include an increase in employer and employee National Insurance contributions from April 2003, an increase in the state retirement age for women from 60 to 65 years, the introduction of stakeholder pensions to increase the share of pensioner income held from private as opposed to public sources, the implementation of reforms as a result of The NHS and

Community Care Act 1990, and the recent decision to provide personal care free at the point of consumption to qualifying individuals in Scotland. Such policy changes have been introduced in order to fund improvements in the quality and access of care for all groups, to enable frail older people to live in their own homes for longer, and to recognize the fiscal implications of increases in the ratio of older people retired from the labour force relative to the population that is economically active.

Concerns over ageing can, however, be traced back over many years. Bauld *et al.* (2000) note that the report of the Royal Commission on Population in 1949 suggested that an ageing population 'might become dangerously unprogressive, falling behind other communities in technical efficiency and economic welfare.' These issues continue to remain high on the policy-makers' agenda today (Royal Commission on Long Term Care 1999; Care Development Group 2001), with questions over the mix of public vs. private funding and concerns over reductions in the number of residential and nursing home beds creating bed-blocking in acute hospital care. The Wanless Report (Wanless 2002) provides the most recent example of the priority given by policy-makers to the implications of ageing for future health and long-term care expenditures.

As a result of the growing policy concerns, it is important to examine critically the assumptions and methods used in studies that measure the projected demographic and disability trends and the implications of such trends for health and long-term care (e.g. social care expenditures) among older people. Each of these issues is considered separately below. The approach is to discuss critical or recent developments in the literature rather than provide a systematic review of all the related literature. The concluding section discusses policy implications and highlights the need and information requirements for further research on the joint relationship between age, disability and long-term care expenditures.

THE RELATIONSHIP BETWEEN AGE AND DISABILITY

Health and social care costs for all people depend not only on life expectancy but also on the proportion of life spent in particular health states (Manton *et al.* 1998). Population ageing driven by improvements in older age mortality will tend to increase costs if life expectancy gains tend to be spent in frailer health states.

THE COMPRESSION OF MORBIDITY HYPOTHESIS

This issue has been the subject of intense debate spanning over two decades. Fries (1980, 1983, 1989; Fries *et al.* 1989) proposed the 'compression of morbidity' hypothesis: the proportion of people surviving to old age will continue to increase, with chronic disease confined to a brief segment towards the end of a fixed biological life span. Fuchs (1984) also assumed an optimistic view that greater life expectancy is associated with reduced morbidity. The contrasting school of thought suggests that greater survival results in people acquiring other diseases, which otherwise would have been avoided had they died (Schneider & Brody 1983; Verbrugge 1984).

Tests of the compression of morbidity hypothesis require empirical data on mortality and morbidity. Mortality data do indeed support the notion of improved survival, often denoted by a rectangularization of the survival curve due to reduced mortality rates at younger ages and consequently more people surviving into older age (OECD 1998b). Yet levels of morbidity or disability are also crucial in determining whether more time in the added life years is being spent in better health. Three points are critical with respect to obtaining good estimates of changes in disability over time: (1) estimates should be standardized to control for changes in the age distribution of the population; (2) estimates should use a valid and broadly recognized measure of disability; and (3) longitudinal survey data that enable tracking cohorts of individuals over time should be used if available.

HEALTHY LIFE EXPECTANCY – METHODOLOGICAL ISSUES

The concept of healthy life expectancy (also known as disability-free life expectancy) is increasingly employed to measure changes in morbidity (Bone *et al*. 1995). This measure estimates the average number of years of life free from disability remaining at particular ages for members of a given population. As such measures are independent of the particular age structure of the population, they directly address the need to standardize for the changing age distribution of the population.

Bone *et al*. (1998) discuss the two methods that are most commonly used to calculate healthy life expectancy. The first is Sullivan's method, which combines data on the incidence of mortality from life tables with data on prevalence of disability over time from repeated cross-sectional surveys (Sullivan 1971). The second approach consists of multistate life-table methods that use longitudinal data on transitions between healthy states to disabled states over time for cohorts of individuals (Schoen 1988). Robine and Mathers (1993) used simulations to show that if transition rates are stable, then the estimates from both methods will be similar. However, if transition rates are changing over time, then the multistate method is preferred, because it directly incorporates specific estimates of transitions between health states.

With either method, it is important to have information on living arrangements, as many surveys only capture the non-institutionalized population. Without adjusting for living arrangements, part of the reason for finding improvements in levels of disability could be due to increased rates of institutionalization (i.e. the less healthy individuals are no longer living in the community) or other supply-side changes in formal care. In the UK context this is of particular importance, given the unprecedented though unsurprising rise in the number of people living in residential and nursing homes in the 1980s and early 1990s (Darton & Wright 1993; Grundy & Glaser 1997).

Measures of healthy life expectancy are useful for comparing population health states between countries and for projecting future trends if consistent definitions of disability are used. It should be noted, however, that researchers such as Williams (1999) are concerned about implicit values inherent in some definitions of disability and therefore advocate broader quality of life measures. The definition of disability and use of longitudinal data are most critical but also most challenging for assessments of trends in healthy life expectancy over time. Measures of disability that have commonly been used range from self-reported disability (e.g. using responses to questions about whether a person is affected by a limiting long-standing illness) to measures of functional impairment to living arrangements.

While self-reports of limiting illness or self-perceived poor health are easily obtained, they are subject to potential reporting bias, as they may vary between respondents with similar conditions who perceive their level of disability differently or over time due to changing societal influences. Measures of functional impairment, such as difficulties in performing independent activities of daily living (IADLs) or activities of daily living (ADLs), are part of a much more standardized assessment. Although the data on such impairment or need for assistance generally result from self-assessment, these measures of functional status have been validated across populations. Institutional residence is generally assumed to be associated with some level of disability and indicates on average a fairly high need for support, though information on variation in impairment among institutionalized persons is difficult to obtain.

Even if the issues about definitions of disability and availability of longitudinal panels over time are addressed, some caution should be exercised when drawing conclusions about health status from national household survey data. Waidmann et al. (1995) discuss trends in self-reported health in the US using data from the National Health Interview Survey. Their findings illustrate the difficulty of drawing conclusions from aggregate trends in health status. They argue that the deterioration in health observed in the 1970s and the subsequent improvement recorded in the following decade may be an artefactual improvement, with the changes related to expansion of income maintenance programmes and earlier diagnosis of pre-existing conditions. They conclude that actual health did not change to the extent observed.

HEALTHY LIFE EXPECTANCY – EMPIRICAL FINDINGS

As a result of the use of longitudinal data and validated measures of disability, Manton and colleagues (Manton et al. 1997, 1998; Manton & Gu 2001) provide some of the most robust evidence of changes in disability among persons aged 65 years or older. These researchers used the National Long Term Care Survey (a longitudinal survey of community-based and institutionalized persons aged 65 and older in the US) from 1982 to 1999. They defined disability as either living in an institutional setting (e.g. nursing home) or having ADL or IADL impairment. Their results indicate a reduction in overall disability of between 0.3 and 0.6 percentage points per year between the early 1980s and the late 1990s, with evidence of an increase in the reduction rate over time.

While Manton and Gu's analysis provides strong evidence of declines in disability for the US and a useful framework for the assessment of changes in disability over time, it is important to determine whether their results are generalizable to other countries. For most countries such as the UK, obtaining comparable estimates is complicated by the lack of longitudinal data and by varying definitions of disability in the available data sets. For example, national household survey evidence from a number of developed countries suggests that, while the proportion of the extra years of life spent in disabled states rose between 1970 and 1990, less time was spent in the most disabled states (Bone et al. 1995; Cambois & Robine 1996; Robine et al. 1997; OECD 1998b). Therefore, healthy life expectancy is not rising as quickly as life expectancy by broad measures of disability, though the proportion of time spent in the most disabled states (which are potentially the most resource-intensive states) is possibly declining.

The UK results were derived primarily from work done by Bone, Bebbington and colleagues (Bone et al. 1998; Bebbington & Comas-Herrera 2000) using Sullivan's methods with the General Household Survey. This survey does not include people living in communal establishments (i.e. the institutionalized population) and the estimates assume a constant disability rate among communal establishments. Table 9.2 summarizes their key results, which show that between 1980 and 1998 life expectancy increased on average each year by 1.7 months and 1.2 months for a 65-year-old male and female, respectively. The corresponding increase for healthy life expectancy free from a

Table 9.2 Average improvement, in months per year, in life expectancy and healthy life expectancy for people at age 65, over the period 1980–1998

	Life expectancy	Healthy life expectancy (time free from limiting long-standing illness)	Healthy life expectancy (ADL impairment-free)
Males	1.7	0.4	1.7
Females	1.2	0.6	1.2

Source: Bebbington and Comas-Herrera (2000), p. 10.

limiting long-standing illness, however, was only 0.4 and 0.6 months on average each year, indicating that healthy life expectancy increased substantially less than life expectancy by this disability measure. Yet healthy life expectancy did increase at the same rate as life expectancy for both males and females for the more severe disability measure of reporting impairment in one or more ADLs. Therefore, whether healthy life expectancy within the UK has been increasing commensurately with life expectancy depends largely on the measure of disability used.

Stearns and Butterworth (2001) used data from two cross-sectional national household surveys, the 1985 OPCS Survey of Disability among Adults in Private Households and the 1996/7 Disability Follow-up Survey to the 1996 Family Resources Survey, to characterize disability trends in Scotland. The definition of disability used was consistent across the two surveys but substantially more inclusive than the definitions used by Manton and colleagues or Bone, Bebbington and colleagues. Since the sampling strategies differed between the two surveys, the methodology is very different from the multistate approach used by Manton and colleagues and also potentially different from the work by Bone, Bebbington and colleagues, in which the survey had an essentially consistent sampling strategy over time. While comparisons across the two surveys or to other studies are problematic due to data and methodological differences, evidence was found of reductions in the proportion of older people in Scotland with disabilities between 1985 and 1997.

THE RELATIONSHIP BETWEEN AGE AND EXPENDITURES

The relationship between age and expenditures is complex. It may be argued that increasing longevity is partly dependent on provision of health and social care, whilst the reverse is also true: the supply of care and associated expenditures are likely to depend on the age distribution of the population. Standard theory of the demand for health under the Grossman model (Grossman 1972) predicts that ageing leads to a reduction in health status and a demand for more care. However, care can improve health and life expectancies and so by itself can contribute to population ageing. In other instances, care may improve life expectancies but have no substantial effects on levels of health status.

CRISIS VS. MANAGEABLE THEORISTS

Demographers, economists, sociologists and other social scientists have projected the impacts of population ageing on the expenditures associated with the health and social care system using a variety of methods. Within this field, Rosenberg (2000) distinguishes between two broad competing schools of thought.

First, the *crisis theorists* (Schneider & Guralnik 1990; Marzouk 1991; Mendelson & Schwartz 1993; Henripin 1994) conclude that growth in the older population generates significant costs for the health and social care system which are not sustainable given current methods of health care organization and finance. Second, the *manageable theorists* (Getzen 1992; Denton & Spencer 1995, 1999) see population ageing having a smaller impact on costs to the health and social care system. The argument is that the growth in the older age population is only one component in the sum of factors that are associated with increases in health and social care expenditures. The implication is that all components need to be addressed in devising policies to preserve current systems of publicly funded universal health and social care services.

The main reason why these theorists arrive at different conclusions relates to the way ageing is modelled. Crisis theorists draw heavily on age and sex-standardized utilization rates and costs, where change over time within countries is driven by changes in the projected size of the older population and increasing proportions of the population in older age groups. One weakness with this approach is that it does not allow for changes in age-related disability or associated health or social care requirements. More importantly, however, no control is made for variables that affect expenditure decisions at the macro level, such as the level and growth of national income.

MANAGEABLE THEORISTS I

It is possible to identify two further broad groups of manageable theorists. The first group combine population projections, utilization and costs alongside other models of the economy, which may include some or all of the following components: labour force participation, capital stock, investment, output, taxes, disposable income, consumption and savings. Their concern is with both *demand*, the ways in which ageing of the population might affect patterns of expenditure (including the demand for publicly provided services), and *supply*, the ways in which it might affect the productive capacity of the economy. The main conclusion from this group is that higher future health care costs are manageable provided there is at least modest economic growth.

Prominent within this field are studies by Denton and Spencer (1995, 1999). They show that when projected expenditures are compared to the projected productive capacity of the economy, total expenditure for all public programmes will be a *smaller* percentage of GDP in 2031 than in 1991. They emphasize that the estimates are dependent on assumptions relating to achieving a reallocation of resources from other publicly funded programmes (such as education expenditures) and savings in health care expenditures resulting from efficiency gains.

MANAGEABLE THEORISTS II

A second group of manageable theorists utilize demographic, health expenditure and income per capita variables for groups of countries, either measured using cross-sectional or time-series data. The theoretical justification for this approach is provided by Getzen (1992, 2001), who argues that extrapolation from higher health care costs per older person to higher national health care costs for an older population suffers from a 'fallacy of composition' (or the assumption that what is true for the individual must be true for the aggregate of individuals). Using regression analysis of growth in national health expenditures against the percentage of the population aged 65 years or over, income per capita and lagged income for 20 countries between 1960 and 1988, Getzen (1992) finds that ageing had no significant relationship with expenditure growth. His conclusion is that whilst greater longevity may increase the demand for care at the individual level of decision-making, the budget constraint at the national level means that health care expenditures are dependent on growth in national income and political choices rather than levels of ill health. In short, the measurement of a macroeconomic variable, such as national health care expenditures, cannot be obtained by simple aggregation across individuals or generalized from micro observations (Getzen 2001).

EMPIRICAL SUPPORT FOR THEORIES – MACRO EVIDENCE

A number of studies in the international comparisons of health care expenditures literature support the work of manageable theorists. O'Connell (1996) concluded that population ageing did not increase per capita health spending amongst 21 OECD countries between 1975 and 1990. In an alternative specification employing country-specific age variables rather than a single age variable, an effect was found for some countries. However, in half of these cases, the sign of the coefficient was negative. Barros (1998) extends the approach by focusing on differences in growth (as opposed to levels) of health care expenditures for 24 OECD countries. He finds no significant relationship between the percentage of the population aged 65 years or over and average per capita health expenditure growth, after controlling for national income and type of health care reimbursement system. These results support the findings of many other econometric studies that consider the association between per capita health care spending and per capita national income after controlling for population age structure and other health system variables (Roberts 1999; Gerdtham & Jonsson 2000).

EMPIRICAL SUPPORT FOR THEORIES – MICRO EVIDENCE

Considering Canadian and US studies, Rosenberg (2000) highlights that evidence supporting the assumptions within manageable theorists' models can be drawn from a number of sources. For example, McDaniel (1987) demonstrates that in the 1970s and 1980s health care costs increased far more rapidly than the older population. While hospital operating expenditures in Canada increased at an annual rate averaging 14.9% between 1961 and 1980, the net effect of changes in the age composition of the population was essentially zero (cited by Marshall 1994, p. 236). Newhouse (1992) calculates that the change in age composition between 1950 and 1987 accounted for only 15% of US expenditure growth. Using data from British Columbia, Barer et al. (1995, p. 218) argue that the disproportionate utilization of health services by the older population is 'driven by changes in patterns of health care practice, not in the numbers and ages of elderly people in the population.' These findings are confirmed in a more recent study by Evans et al. (2001). They find major discrepancies between age-based forecasts of acute inpatient hospital days, physician fee per item of service reimbursements, pharmaceutical expenditures and actual use or expenditures between 1969 and 2000. This study demonstrates the weaknesses of simple linear extrapolations and the sensitivity of projections to assumptions made regarding age and sex-specific utilization rates and costs.

OTHER EXPENDITURE DETERMINANTS – PROXIMITY TO DEATH

An emerging body of literature suggests that the relationship between age and expenditures depends on the extent to which age relative to time until death is associated with health care expenditures. Projections of future expenditures based on age without accounting for age at death may overestimate the effect of improved life expectancy on costs.

Several studies attempt to answer this question by comparing the proportion of total expenditures accounted for in the last year of life by the proportion who died (Lubitz & Prihoda 1984; Kovar 1986), or by estimating resource use close to death with resource use farther away from death (McCall 1984; Lubitz & Riley 1993; van Weel & Michels 1997).

These studies, however, do not provide evidence of the strength of the relationship between expenditures, proximity to death and age, as they do not control for both age and time until death in estimating expenditure (Norton 2000). Studies employing such designs (Lubitz et al. 1995; McNamee et al. 1999; Zweifel et al. 1999; McGrail et al. 2000; Yang et al. 2002) show that age has little or no effect on expenditures after adjusting for remaining life expectancy. Lubitz et al. (1995) found that Medicare expenditures rose rapidly in the three years prior to death, but less so for older persons. McNamee et al.

(1999) found that health and social care expenditures among frail older people were significantly associated with proximity to death, with age displaying no significant relationship. Zweifel *et al.* (1999) showed that age had no independent effect on health care expenditures after adjusting for remaining life expectancy. In one of the first studies that compared health and social care costs, McGrail *et al.* (2000) estimated that health care costs declined with rising age for those who died, but that nursing and social care costs rose. Using data from the US Medicare programme, Yang *et al.* (2002) show that time to death is the main reason for higher inpatient care expenditures, while ageing is the main reason for higher long-term care expenditures. The implication from these studies is that expenditures are not necessarily affected by population ageing. Rather, an increase in the proportion of older people in the total population shifts a substantial amount of expenditures to higher ages, especially hospital expenditures.

With the exception of McNamee *et al.* (1999), McGrail *et al.* (2000) and Yang *et al.* (2002), a weakness in most of these studies is that they focus on acute hospital use due to lack of data on long-term care use. This drawback may be major, as total costs include those incurred both in acute hospital care settings and those health and social care costs incurred in community and residential/nursing home settings. For example, Spillman and Lubitz (2000) show that long-term care expenditures increase at an increasing rate for older persons. The rise in nursing home costs within the US with age at death is sufficient to counteract the moderating effect of declining Medicare expenditures, so that the rate of increase in total spending from the age of 65 years until death also rises with age at death.

CONCLUSIONS

Evidence of the relationship between population ageing and disability is mixed. Whilst among older individuals there is a positive relationship between higher age and greater disability (Stuck *et al.* 1999), it is less clear whether population ageing necessarily results in greater disability in the population. Empirical evidence has failed to resolve this ambiguity at least in part because of the use of different measures of disability in different surveys. In addition, interpretation may also be more difficult because of the requirement to use cut-off points to define disability prevalence in measurement of healthy life expectancy estimates. Any heterogeneity in the thresholds used will mean that comparisons between studies cannot be made for the purposes of identifying trends. Further, such measures may be insensitive to changes in levels of disability severity above the thresholds used to define disability. For these reasons, it is difficult to conclude from most studies whether the greater numbers of older people in the future will be healthier than current cohorts.

Examination of the relationship between ageing and expenditures also reveals a complex pattern. A number of cross-sectional and panel data studies within and between countries show that age has little or no effect on expenditures once adjustment is made for other characteristics of individuals, care providers or health care systems. However, emerging longitudinal studies on effects of proximity to death relative to age *per se* show the importance of distinguishing between these effects in predictions of health *and* social care expenditures. Therefore, greater numbers of people surviving to older ages may result in higher total (health and social care) expenditures, but not to the extent predicted by age alone. A weakness in most of these studies is that health status is not measured. An important research priority therefore is to examine the relationship between the age structure of populations, levels of disability and total expenditure patterns on health and social care between different countries.

POLICY IMPLICATIONS WITHIN THE UK

As estimates of trends in disability and healthy life expectancy are dependent in part on the definitions of disability used and survey design, policy decisions over these factors are likely to be critical for projections of the cost implications of caring for older people. In estimating the costs of long-term care, the Royal Commission on Long Term Care (1999) assumed constant health expectancy levels for the elderly over the next 50 years. As part of a sensitivity analysis, the report considered alternately a 1% increase and decrease in age-specific dependency rates. Costs under the 1% increase were substantially higher, while under the scenario of reductions in dependency, the estimated costs of providing free personal care were roughly halved during the period 1995 and 2051 (Royal Commission on Long Term Care 1999). As the results are very sensitive to assumptions regarding disability levels, policy-makers need to ensure that decisions are based on the best available data, ideally from longitudinal surveys that track changes in validated measures of health status.

As highlighted in the Wanless Report (Wanless 2002), an additional factor concerning policy-makers relates to the role of patient expectations. An assumption is made that people expect better quality care, measured in terms of faster access to services, reductions in care inequalities and use of the latest available technology. In terms of health care delivery, policy-makers have already responded to rising expectations through the introduction of National Service Frameworks and the National Institute for Clinical Excellence (NICE). Should these policies be successful, more older people will receive health care. One specific example in this context is the NICE policy guidance on prescribing new therapies for Alzheimer's disease, which states that all patients with a particular level of cognitive impairment are eligible for treatment (NICE 2001).

In the field of social or long-term care, a number of legislative changes have been introduced. The abolition of user charges for personal care in Scotland beginning in 2002 may increase the propensity to seek care, although the policy was only implemented because any associated increase in expenditures was estimated to be affordable. Existing charges for personal care in England and Wales may increase demand for a similar policy response. Proposals aimed at improving carer welfare, such as implementation of the Carers and Disabled Children Act 2000, indicate that policy-makers are prioritizing the role of informal carers (Hirst 2001; Parker 2002). For example, the policy of 'carer-blind services' aims to ensure that service assessment is based on levels of disability, irrespective of whether older people co-reside with a carer. Concerns also remain, however, over long-term care provision by the formal sector. Recent reductions in the supply of places in residential and nursing homes may lead to bed-blocking and greater expenditures in acute hospital care (Wanless 2002). Policy-makers may therefore need to develop incentives to encourage care providers to remain in the long-term care market.

FUTURE RESEARCH DIRECTIONS

A factor limiting rigorous analysis of the relationships between ageing and disability, ageing and expenditures, and the joint relationship between these factors is the lack in many countries of longitudinal panel surveys. At present there is no national longitudinal data source in the UK to allow measurement of trends in disability among older people (Bone et al. 1998). Most analyses rely on cross-sectional General Household Survey data, which only sample those resident in private households. The Health Survey for England conducted in 2000 (Department of Health 2002) included for the first time a survey of the health of older people in care homes, so these data could be used to refine estimates of the level of disability among people in institutional settings.

An alternative to using broadly comprehensive household surveys is to use longitudinal data collected within specific populations. One possibility could be sources such as the Cognitive Function and Ageing Study (http://www.mrc-bsu.cam.ac.uk/cfas/new2/index.htm). This study is a multicentre age-stratified randomized survey of 10,377 individuals aged 65 years or over resident in private households or institutions. At present, cross-sectional analyses of these data provide a profile of current levels of physical and mental disability (MRC CFAS and RIS MRC CFAS 1999; MRC CFAS 2001) and estimates of future years of disabled life (MRC CFAS 2000). Further analyses to exploit the longitudinal nature of the data remain possible, with the potential to produce estimates using multistate methods. Yet even this survey may not be sufficiently comprehensive, as the study is only currently collecting limited data on measures of health and social care utilization. Until a more comprehensive NHS information system is available, it would be extremely useful if such studies could be extended to gather more complete measures of the use of health and social care.

Finally, several areas relevant to the assessment of the relationships between age, disability and expenditures have not been discussed in this chapter. Two in particular deserve attention. First, the economic resources of older people may be an important determinant of both levels of disability and care expenditures (Almond *et al.* 1999). Future cohorts may well be wealthier on average in retirement than current groups of older people, due to higher levels of home ownership and membership of occupational pension schemes, although inequalities may also increase (Evandrou & Falkingham 2000). Second, the availability of informal care has been shown to be a significant variable in the demand for formal care (McNamee *et al.* 1999). Informal care by spouses is likely to be an increasing source of support to frail older people in the future, due to reductions in male mortality (Pickard *et al.* 2000). In addition, other policies such as implementation of free personal care in Scotland may affect the supply of informal care. As empirical evidence relating to the magnitude of substitution between formal and informal care for personal care services is limited, this policy development presents an ideal opportunity to assess the response of informal carers. The effects of changes in wealth or availability of informal care would be likely to shift any predictions of future expenditures for long-term care (Wittenberg *et al.* 2001). Further research on these issues facilitated by longitudinal panels including standardized measures of disability and measures of health and social care use remain a priority.

ACKNOWLEDGEMENTS

Support for this chapter was provided in part by the NHS Executive Northern and Yorkshire Region and by the Scottish Executive Health Department. We are grateful for the comments of David Torgerson on a previous draft. The authors are responsible for the information presented, and the views expressed in the chapter should not be construed to belong to the funding sources.

REFERENCES

Almond S, Bebbington A, Judge K, Mangalore R and O'Donnell O (1999) *Poverty, Disability, and the Use of Long-Term Care Services*. The Royal Commission on Long-Term Care. Stationery Office, London.

Barer ML, Evans RG and Hertzman C (1995) Avalanche or glacier: health care and the demographic rhetoric. *Canadian Journal on Aging*, **14**, 193–224.

Barros P (1998) The black box of health care expenditure growth determinants. *Health Economics*, **7**, 533–544.

Bauld L, Chesterman J, Davies B, Judge K and Mangalore R (2000) *Caring for Older People: an Assessment of Community Care in the 1990s.* Ashgate, Aldershot.

Bebbington A and Comas-Herrera A (2000) *Healthy Life Expectancy: Trends to 1998, and the implications for long term care costs.* PSSRU Discussion Paper 1695, www.ukc.ac.uk/PSSRU, December.

Bone M, Bebbington A, Jagger C, Morgan K and Nicolas G (1995) *Health Expectancy and Its Uses.* HMSO, London.

Bone M, Bebbington A and Nicolas G (1998) Policy applications of health expectancy. *Journal of Aging and Health*, **10**, 136–153.

Cambois E and Robine J (1996) An international comparison of trends in disability free life expectancy. In R Eisen and F Sloan (Eds), *Long-term Care: Economic Issues and Policy Solutions.* Kluwer, Dordrecht.

Care Development Group (2001) *Providing Free Personal Care for Older People: Research Commissioned to Inform the Work of the Care Development Group.* Edited by Diane Machin and Danny McShane. Scottish Executive Central Research Unit, www.scotland.gov.uk/cru/kd01/red/pfpc-00.asp.

Cutler D and Meara E (2001) *Changes in the age distribution of mortality over the 20th century.* NBER Working Paper Series, 8556. National Bureau of Economic Research.

Darton R and Wright K (1993) Changes in the provision of long-stay care. *Health and Social Care in the Community*, **1**, 11–25.

Denton F and Spencer B (1995) Demographic change and the cost of publicly funded health care. *Canadian Journal on Aging*, **14**, 174–192.

Denton F and Spencer B (1999) *Population aging and its economic costs: a survey of the issues and evidence.* SEDAP Research Paper No. 1.

Department of Health (2002) Website accessed on 17 June 2002: http://www.official-documents.co.uk/document/deps/doh/survey00/hse00.htm.

Department of Health (2001) *National Service Framework for Older People.* Department of Health, London.

Evandrou M and Falkingham J (2000) Looking back to look forward: lessons from four birth cohorts for ageing in the 21st century. *Population Trends*, **99**, 21–30.

Evans RG, McGrail KM, Morgan SG, Barer ML and Hertzman C (2001) Apocalypse no: population aging and the future of health care systems. *Canadian Journal on Aging*, **20**, 160–191.

Fries J (1980) Aging, natural death and the compression of morbidity. *New England Journal of Medicine*, **303**, 130–135.

Fries J (1983) The compression of morbidity. *Milbank Memorial Fund Quarterly*, **61**, 397–419.

Fries J (1989) The compression of morbidity: near or far? *The Milbank Quarterly*, **67**, 208–232.

Fries J, Green L and Levine S (1989) Health promotion and the compression of morbidity. *The Lancet*, **1**(8636), 481–483.

Fuchs V (1984) Though much is taken: reflections on aging, health and medical care. *Milbank Memorial Fund Quarterly*, **62**, 142–166.

Gerdtham UG and Jonsson B (2000) International comparisons of health expenditure. In AJ Culyer and J Newhouse (Eds), *Handbook of Health Economics.* Elsevier, Amsterdam.

Getzen T (1992) Population ageing and the growth of health expenditures. *Journal of Gerontology: Social Sciences*, **47**, S98–104.

Getzen T (2001) Aging and health care expenditures: a comment on Zweifel, Felder and Meiers. *Health Economics*, **10**, 175–177.

Grossman M (1972) On the concept of health capital and the demand for health. *Journal of Political Economy*, **80**, 223–255.

Grundy E and Glaser K (1997) Trends in, and transitions to, institutional residence among older people in England and Wales. *Journal of Epidemiology and Community Health*, **51**, 531–540.

Henripin J (1994) The financial consequences of aging. *Canadian Public Policy*, **20**, 78–94.

Hirst M (2001) Trends in informal care in Great Britain during the 1990s. *Health and Social Care in the Community*, **9**, 348–357.

Kovar M (1986) Expenditures for the medical care of elderly people living in the community in 1980. *The Milbank Quarterly*, **64**, 100–132.

Lubitz J and Prihoda R (1984) The use and costs of Medicare services in the last two years of life. *Health Care Financing Review*, **5**, 117–131.

Lubitz J and Riley G (1993) Trends in Medicare payments in the last year of life. *New England Journal of Medicine*, **328**, 1092–1096.

Lubitz J, Beebe J and Baker C (1995) Longevity and Medicare expenditures. *New England Journal of Medicine*, **332**, 999–1003.

Manton K and Gu X (2001) Changes in the prevalence of chronic disability in the United States black and nonblack population above age 65 from 1982 to 1999. *Proceedings of the National Academy of Sciences*, **98**, 6354–6359.

Manton K, Corder L and Stallard E (1997) Chronic disability trends in elderly United States populations: 1982–1994. *Proceedings of the National Academy of Sciences*, **94**, 2593–2598.

Manton K, Stallard E and Corder L (1998) Economic effects of reducing disability. *American Economic Review*, **88**, 101–105.

Marshall V (1994) *Aging in Canada: Social Perspectives*. Fitzhenry and Whiteside, Toronto.

Marzouk M (1991) Aging, age-specific health care costs and the future health care burden in Canada. *Canadian Public Policy*, **17**, 490–506.

McCall N (1984) Utilization and costs of Medicare services by beneficiaries in their last year of life. *Medical Care*, **22**, 329–342.

McDaniel S (1987) Demographic aging as a guiding paradigm in Canada's welfare state. *Canadian Public Policy*, **13**, 330–336.

McGrail K, Green B, Barer ML, Evans RG, Hertzman C and Normand C (2000) Age, costs of acute and long-term care and proximity to death: evidence for 1987–88 and 1994–95 in British Columbia. *Age and Ageing*, **29**, 249–253.

McLoughlin J (1991) *The Demographic Revolution*. Faber and Faber, London.

McNamee P, Gregson B, Buck D, Bamford C, Bond J, Wright K (1999) Costs of formal care for frail older people in England: the resource implications study of the MRC cognitive function and ageing study. *Social Science and Medicine*, **48**, 331–341.

Mendelson D and Schwartz W (1993) Effects of aging and population growth on health care costs. *Health Affairs*, **12**, 119–125.

MRC CFAS and RIS MRC CFAS (1999) Medical Research Council Cognitive Function and Ageing Study and Resource Implications Study. Profile of disability in elderly people: estimates from a longitudinal population study. *British Medical Journal*, **318**, 1108–1111.

MRC CFAS (2000) Medical Research Council Cognitive Function and Ageing Study. Socioeconomic status and the expectation of disability in old age: estimates for England. *Journal of Epidemiology and Community Health*, **54**, 286–292.

MRC CFAS (2001) Medical Research Council Cognitive Function and Ageing Study. Health and ill-health in the older population in England and Wales. *Age and Ageing*, **30**, 53–62.

Newhouse J (1992) Medical care costs: how much welfare loss? *Journal of Economic Perspectives*, **6**, 3–22.

NICE (National Institute for Clinical Excellence) (2001). *Guidance on the use of donepezil, rivastigmine and galantamine for the treatment of Alzheimer's Disease.* Technology Appraisal Guidance No. 19.

Norton E (2000) Long term care. In AJ Culyer and J Newhouse (Eds), *Handbook of Health Economics.* Elsevier, Amsterdam.

O'Connell J (1996) The relationship between health expenditures and the age structure of the population in OECD countries. *Health Economics*, **5**, 573–578.

OECD (1996) *Caring for Frail Elderly People: Policies in Evolution.* Organisation for Economic Co-operation and Development, Paris.

OECD (1998a) *Maintaining Prosperity in an Ageing Society.* Organisation for Economic Co-operation and Development, Paris.

OECD (1998b) *The health of older persons in OECD countries: is it improving fast enough to compensate for population ageing?* Labour Market and Social Policy Paper No. 37. Organisation for Economic Co-operation and Development, Paris.

OECD (2000) *Reforms for an Ageing Society.* Organisation for Economic Co-operation and Development, Paris.

Parker G (2002) 10 years of the new community care: good in parts? *Health and Social Care in the Community*, **10**, 1–5.

Pickard L, Wittenberg R, Comas-Herrera A, Davies B and Darton R (2000) Relying on informal care in the new century? Informal care for elderly people in England to 2031. *Ageing and Society*, **20**, 745–772.

Raleigh VS (1997) The demographic timebomb. *British Medical Journal*, **315**, 442–443.

Roberts J (1999) Sensitivity of elasticity estimates for OECD health care spending: analysis of a dynamic heterogeneous data field. *Health Economics*, **8**, 459–472.

Robine JM and Mathers CD (1993) Measuring the compression or expansion of morbidity through changes in healthy life expectancy. In JM Robine, CD Mathers, MR Bone and J Romieu (Eds), *Calculation of Health Expectancies: Harmonization, Consensus Achieved and Future Perspectives.* John Libbey, Eurotext, London.

Robine J, Romieu I and Cambois E (1997) Health expectancies and current research. *Reviews in Clinical Gerontology*, **7**, 73–81.

Rosenberg M (2000) *The effects of ageing on the Canadian health care system.* SEDAP Research Paper No. 14.

Royal Commission on Long Term Care (1999) *With respect to old age: long term care – rights and responsibilities.* Stationery Office, London.

Schneider EL and Brody JA (1983) Aging, natural death, and the compression of morbidity – another view. *New England Journal of Medicine*, **309**, 854–856.

Schneider E and Guralnik J (1990) The aging of America: impact on health care costs. *Journal of the American Medical Association*, **263**, 2335–2340.

Schoen R (1988) Practical uses of multistate population models. *Annual Review of Sociology*, **14**, 341–361.

Spillman B and Lubitz J (2000) The effect of longevity on spending for acute and long-term care. *New England Journal of Medicine*, **342**, 1409–1415.

Stearns SC and Butterworth S (2001) Demand for and utilisation of personal care services for the elderly. In D Machin and D McShane (Eds), *Providing Free Personal Care for Older People: Research Commissioned to Inform the Work of the Care*

Development Group. Scottish Executive Central Research Unit, www.scotland.gov. uk/cru/kd01/red/pfpc-00.asp.

Stuck A, Walthert J, Nikolaus T, Bula C, Wehmann C and Beck J (1999) Risk factors for functional status decline in community-living elderly: a systematic literature review. *Social Science and Medicine*, **48**, 445–469.

Sullivan DE (1971) A single index of mortality and morbidity. *HMSA Health Report*, **86**, 347–354.

van Weel C and Michels J (1997) Dying, not old age, to blame for costs of health care. *The Lancet*, **350**, 1159–1160.

Verbrugge L (1984) Longer life but worsening health – trends in health and mortality of middle-aged and older persons. *Milbank Memorial Fund Quarterly*, **62**, 475–519.

Waidmann T, Bound J and Schoenbaum M (1995) The illusion of failure: trends in the self-reported health of the US elderly. *The Milbank Quarterly*, **73**, 253–287.

Wanless D (2002) *Securing our future health: taking a long term view*. HM Treasury, London.

Williams A (1999) Calculating the global burden of disease: time for a strategic reappraisal? *Health Economics*, **8**, 1–8.

Wittenberg R, Pickard L, Comas-Herrera A, Davies B and Darton R (2001) Demand for long-term care for older people in England to 2031. *Health Statistics Quarterly*, **12**, 5–17.

World Bank (1999) *World Development Indicators*. Washington D.C., World Bank.

Yang Z, Norton EC and Stearns SC (2002) Longevity and health care expenditures: the real reasons older people spend more. *Journal of Gerontology* (forthcoming).

Zweifel P, Felder S and Meiers M (1999) Ageing of population and health care expenditure: a red herring? *Health Economics*, **8**, 485–496.

10

Economic Challenges in Primary Care

ALAN MAYNARD
York Health Policy Group, University of York

ANTHONY SCOTT
Health Economics Research Unit, University of Aberdeen

INTRODUCTION

Primary care is regarded by some as the 'cornerstone' of any well-designed health care system (Bloor *et al.* 2000). It is usually defined as being the first point of contact for patients seeking health care, as offering longitudinal responsibility for patients, and as providing integration of physical, psychological and social aspects of health care (Starfield 1998). In the UK National Health Service (NHS), primary care has traditionally been seen as a system of care managed and largely operated by general practitioners (GPs) who are the first point of contact for upwards of 95% of patients, and who act as 'gatekeepers' to the hospital system. The words 'system' and 'managed' infer both a 'set of connected parts' and control respectively. Primary care in the NHS is largely delivered by a collection of self-employed entrepreneurs who nonetheless receive all of their income and resources from the NHS. They provide services to patients in which activity, outcomes and access vary along a number of dimensions (Seddon *et al.* 2001).

Performance is difficult to measure as the system is largely free of integrated information systems and so is also difficult to manage because of the traditional 'independent contractor' (self-employed) status of practitioners. Whilst some groups of primary care suppliers now have the information technology to measure and monitor process and activity in primary care, the IT system is not integrated regionally or nationally and is not usually a central element in patient and system management. Furthermore there is little measurement of outcomes both in terms of the proficiency of practitioners to

Advances in Health Economics. Edited by Anthony Scott, Alan Maynard and Robert Elliott.
© 2003 John Wiley & Sons, Ltd

whom primary care patients are referred for diagnostic and inpatient hospital care, and in terms of benefits to patients in primary care settings. Ideally, both mortality and quality of life outcomes would be measured for patient episodes with integration of primary and secondary care data. Unfortunately such data are not available for practitioners, managers or patients.

Nevertheless, the lack of data has not prevented major structural reforms in the NHS. These have given primary care a more central role in resource allocation decisions, particularly in England with Primary Care Trusts replacing health authorities as the main commissioners of health care. When coupled with the recent unprecedented increases in NHS expenditure, which is forecast to rise from 6.5% to over 8.2% of GDP by 2008 (HM Treasury 2002), it seems likely that the decisions made by primary care managers and practitioners will have a major influence on how these extra resources are spent across the NHS.

In this chapter, the central economic issues in this ongoing debate will be reviewed critically and with reference to the current state of knowledge. Both supply and demand-side issues in primary care will be examined. In the first section the issues around workforce recruitment and retention are discussed and this is complemented by a review of the literature about nurse–doctor substitution. A central issue in recruitment and retention is the nature of the employment contract and the systems of remuneration used to reward practitioners. This is discussed in the third section. Demand-side issues are then reviewed both in terms of continuing policy advocacy of contentious reforms such as user charges for GP services, and in terms of issues related to access such as the cross-elasticities of demand between existing and new forms of patient care (e.g. NHS Direct, 'walk in centres', hospital Accident and Emergency facilities, and GP out-of-hours services). A final section reviews the policy and research challenges faced by primary care in the next decade.

WORKFORCE

Employment trends suggest that recruitment and retention of GPs is a major problem. Figure 10.1 shows that there were fewer GPs aged under 35 years in 2000 compared to 1990, suggesting that either fewer are entering general practice, or that doctors are delaying their entry into general practice until they are older (Elliott *et al.* 2002). This may also reflect a demand for more flexible working including career breaks or raising families. The demand for flexible working practices means that those GPs that do enter general practice are also more likely to enter on a part-time basis, for both men and women. The proportion of GP Principals who work part time has increased from 5% in 1990 to 16% in 2000. Within this, the proportion of female GPs working part time has more than doubled over the period from 16% in 1990 to 35% in 2000.

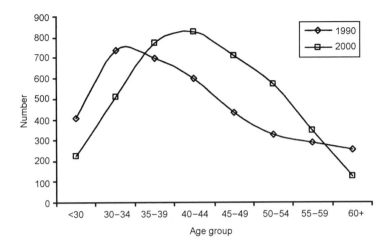

Figure 10.1. Changes in the age distribution of GPs, 1990 and 2000 (Scotland).

This is primarily due to part-time joiners exceeding part-time leavers, rather than an increase in the numbers 'stepping down' to part-time working from full-time working. These trends have also been influenced by an increase in the proportion of female GPs from 29% in 1990 to 39% in 2000 (Elliott *et al.* 2002).

A main feature of a GP's working life during the 1990s was the 24-hour responsibility for the care of their patients. However, since 1995 when major changes were made to the provision of out-of-hours care, many GPs have elected to delegate provision to new out-of-hours organizations. The new GP contract to be introduced in 2003 removes the statutory responsibility for the 24-hour care of patients, with this responsibility transferred to the primary care organization. These changes will further reduce GPs' supply of hours to the NHS and may erode the alleged but unevaluated advantages of continuity of care. The potential benefit is the changes to GPs' 'work–life' balance that is likely to enhance the attractiveness of general practice as a career and enable GPs to provide higher quality of care during the day.

Retention of GPs is also important. Although surveys suggest that the proportion of GPs intending to quit is increasing, there are few data on actual quit rates over time. The exception is Sibbald *et al.* (2002) who show that the proportion of GPs expressing a strong intention to quit rose from 14% in 1998 to 21% in 2001. The main issue with retention is the retirement of GPs. Figure 10.1 shows that there were fewer GPs aged over 60 years in 2000, and that the numbers approaching retirement age are increasing. This is revealed in the shape of the age distribution for those aged 50 years or more in 2000. Interestingly, however, although the number reaching retirement age is likely to increase, there has been no obvious trend in the proportion of GPs aged over 55 years who have left the NHS during the 1990s, suggesting that the propensity to retire has not increased (Elliott *et al.* 2002). Impending pension reform is likely to have a strong effect on retirement decisions.

An important avenue for further research is to examine why these changes are happening so policy can be designed to address them. Part of this research involves examining the relative impact of pecuniary and non-pecuniary factors on decisions to join and leave general practice. There is no empirical evidence which would enable the identification of the factors influencing the relative attractiveness of general practice as a career compared to other careers or other specialties within medicine. There are no data on patterns of individual GP's participation, actual hours of work and earnings so it is not possible to estimate formal labour supply models. Such models would examine the impact of earnings and other factors (personal and job characteristics) on participation and hours worked. Several studies have used stated preference techniques to examine the relative importance of factors influencing job choices for GPs. Studies by Scott (2001) and Gosden *et al.* (2000), which surveyed UK and London GPs respectively, used discrete choice experiments to examine the relative importance of job characteristics in job choice. Scott (2001) found that out-of-hours care was the most important attribute, whereas Gosden *et al.* (2000) showed that GPs in London were most averse to working in areas of high deprivation.

There are two significant ways in which recruitment and retention problems can be mitigated: the use of differing delivery structures, in particular using nurses as substitutes for GPs in a carefully developed triage system, and changes in the contract of employment to make general practice more attractive as a career.

NURSE-DOCTOR SUBSTITUTION

General practice is complex because of the difficulty of sifting the wheat (complex and well-disguised cases) from the chaff of everyday illnesses. Many disease patterns do not require high levels of expertise to manage but do require particular skills in identifying the symptoms and using triage techniques to ensure that the more complex cases are referred on to those with the appropriate expertise. Thus, in principle, appropriately trained nurses can be effective gatekeepers to the primary care system. Furthermore, given speed of practice, working hours and the desire for control of remuneration inflation as they carry out more complex work, nurse practitioners may also be cost-effective substitutes for GPs.

Despite these problems the skill mix used to deliver primary care in the UK has altered significantly. In 1998 there were 36,283 GPs and the doctor population ratio was 1 to 1770, compared with 1 to 1856 in 1988. Over this same period, total support staff in England rose by 82% to 61,331. Practice nurse numbers increased over this period from 3480 to 10,358 and administrative and clerical grade staffing rose from 24,556 to 48,885 (Office of Health Economics 2000, 4.11 and 4.13).

However the evidence about the effectiveness (e.g. do nurses provide the same or better outcomes for patients than doctors carrying out the same tasks?) and cost-effectiveness (e.g. are the patient outcomes as good or better, at less or the same cost?) is poor. There is literature from many countries, but this is limited in quantity, scope and design (Richardson *et al.* 1998). A more recent systematic review found that patient satisfaction was higher for nurses, who also made more investigations and had longer consultations. No differences were found in health status, prescriptions or referrals (Horrocks *et al.* 2002). This study's focus excluded economic variables and, as a consequence, is an incomplete guide to policy choices.

A randomized controlled trial in the USA (Mundinger *et al.* 2000) compared outcomes for patients randomly allocated to doctors and nurse practitioners for follow-up in primary care after an emergency department or urgent care visit. The sample size was over 1300 and outcomes were measured in terms of satisfaction, health status (SF-36) and other tests after 6 months and service utilization after 12 months. The results of the study showed no differences in outcomes or utilization between the two types of provider.

Subsequent discussion of this paper has revealed two problems. Firstly, although the design and execution of this trial is internally valid, it is not externally valid or generalizable because of the unique features of the population included in it (Sox 2000). Secondly, like so many well-designed trials, the authors failed to complete their analysis with a costing to demonstrate the relative cost-effectiveness of the options.

Worldwide and in UK primary care too, new clinical tasks are being taken up by nurses and other non-medically trained personnel. But is this substitution or the development of complements? In principle the increased stock of nurses in general practice should have permitted an increase in the GP population list size. In fact during the last 15 years when nurses have increased in number in general practice the list size has continued to decline. Since the 1990 GP Contract with its greater emphasis and rewards for immunization, vaccination, cervical cytology and monitoring of the health status of the over 75s and health promotion, GPs have increasingly delegated these tasks to nurses. In principle the time freed could have led to either more consultations and/or longer consultations, but there is no evidence this happened (Office of Health Economics 2000, table 4.1; Bloor & Maynard 2001).

The policy issue is whether the driver for increased non-GP staffing in the primary care sector represents substitution or complementarity at work. The evidence from the United States seems unambiguous.

In the early 1990s it was confidently predicted that managed care would not only drive down the fees of physicians but also lead to the eradication of excess medical staffing in the US health care system. In part this was to be achieved by substitution of nurse practitioners for physicians (Weiner 1991). By the late 1990s it was evident that not only was there no surplus of US physicians (predicted earlier to be in excess of 100,000 by the end of the century), but there was also a large increase in what the Americans call 'non-physician assistants' (NPAs) (Cooper *et al.* 1998). The number of NPAs, 228,000 in 1995, was predicted to rise to 384,000 in 2005; a growth rate twice that of physicians and with most of the new staff going into primary care.

Thus the UK equivalent of NPAs may not be substitutes for GPs but complements. The interesting consequence of this is that the virtual monopoly of doctors as the principal providers of and gatekeepers to health care is being eroded. However, given the growth rates of nurse and other staffing in primary care, what are complements now could become substitutes in the future. The ambitious growth in UK medical school intakes could then lead to a doctor surplus within 10 years, with GPs clawing back tasks now carried out by nurses.

The benefit of the rapid growth in the number of nurses and other staff used in primary care has a poor evidence base. This unevaluated social experiment is now being complemented by a rapid and significant development of nurse prescribing. The English Secretary of State for Health has indicated that nurses are likely to be able to prescribe most pharmaceuticals in the near future. He insisted that such prescribing would mean that there would be 'no formulary, no restricted list of drugs and no restriction on the dose or type of prescribing' (Horton 2002).

At present there are 23,000 nurse prescribers in the NHS, and this number will grow to 30,000 in 2004. However, whilst such practitioners may have considerable skills, they, like pharmacists who also wish to have enhanced prescribing roles, have little training in diagnostic skills. Many patients in primary care are old with complex co-morbidities and the potential risks of poor diagnosis and inappropriate prescribing are considerable. Horton (2002) has argued for careful evaluation with prescribing pilots. This work might focus on identifying efficient means of creating diagnostic skills as well as randomized trials of the comparative performance of doctors, nurses and pharmacists in the delivery of cost-effective pharmaceutical care.

Perhaps prescribing will change radically in the next decade? Market research in the USA, Germany, France and Japan shows that the majority of the population believe both that pharmaceutical companies should be allowed to provide information directly to consumers on the internet and that it is likely that consumers will be able to purchase prescription medicines on the internet without visiting a doctor (Harris Interactive 2002). The effects of such liberalization on expenditure and efficiency are unknown.

THE PRIMARY CARE CONTRACT

A main factor that influences the supply of GPs, as well as their performance and behaviour, is the employment contract. In the UK, GPs have been paid through a mix of capitation, fee-for-service, and flat rate payments. Robinson's (2001) appraisal of theory and practice in the design of physician payment systems opens as follows: 'there are many mechanisms for paying physicians; some are good and some are bad. The three worst are fee for service, capitation and salary.' His point is that such systems alone generate behaviours inconsistent with the provision of good access to high-quality health care. As a consequence these payment systems have to be diluted with elements of rival payment systems, what Robinson calls blended remuneration.

The failures of the simple systems are usually depicted as follows, although the evidence base tends to be casual rather than systematically derived from well designed and executed trials. Capitation leads to 'shirking' as practitioners avoid the chronically ill and dump patients who may be high cost and who generate high levels of hospital referrals. Fee-for-service rewards over-provision and the delivery of inappropriate services, can induce fraudulent claims and necessitate the need to police practitioners and may create what American researchers call 'churning' or cross-referrals to colleagues to generate income. Salary payment is expected to reduce productivity by generating on-the-job leisure (e.g. the consumption of inappropriate continuous medical education rather than caring for patients) and induce 'passing the buck' where possible. A recent systematic review of payments for primary care physicians found only six well-controlled studies (Gosden *et al.* 2001). Evidence of behaviour change was found, some of which supports the stylized hypotheses above, although it was difficult to generalize results across settings. The evidence does not, however, focus on the effect of payment systems on recruitment and retention.

The dominant national employment contract for GPs in the UK is unusual in that GPs have had 'independent contractor' status in exchange for agreeing to provide comprehensive care for the patients on their list for every day of the year. Whilst self-employed status offers some tax advantages, it is characterized by vagueness in the meaning of comprehensive care. This gives GPs some discretion over the nature of their work. The great variation in practice access and activity was highlighted in the 1980s when a report revealed that GPs in one area were in contact with the patients on their list for less than 30 hours per week on average (Wilkin & Metcalf 1984). The contract, which bound the GP to provide care within the NHS, required that they render those services generally provided under the heading of 'General Medical Services'. Such circularity led to this arrangement being dubbed the John Wayne contract: 'a GP's got to do what a GP's got to do!' (Maynard & Dowson 1985).

This contract with its flexibility gave practitioners opportunities to vary their practices and this was very attractive to a profession which was largely male. However the increasing gender change in the staffing of general practice, together with increasing demands also by male practitioners not to be 'on call' and covering nights and weekends, has led to contract reform.

The 1990 contract reform was designed to improve the management of primary care, and provide specific incentives for GPs to provide health promotion and preventive services, while also making them more responsive to their patients. The problems of the contract had been obvious for some years but difficult to tackle due to the opposition of the trade union, the British Medical Association. Thus the government in 1986 wanted to 'raise the general quality of these services nearer to that of the best' and recognizing the great variation in access and processes of care, to reward better service provision with a 'good practice allowance'. It also sought to make practitioners more responsive to consumers by raising the proportion of the average GP's remuneration from capitation from 45 to 60% of the total (Department of Social Security 1986).

These proposals were not implemented due to the profession's opposition and when a frustrated junior Minister from 1986 returned to the Department of Health as Secretary of State in 1990, he imposed the new contract on the profession. The objective was to define core tasks and induce appropriate performance by financial incentives. The target level of GP remuneration from capitation was increased to 60%, although there has been no evidence that this has made GPs more responsive to patients' needs as was hoped.

Fees per item of service were revised and developed firstly to encourage higher levels of coverage in areas such as immunization and vaccination, and cervical cytology, and secondly to encourage activity in new areas of service provision such as minor surgery, screening of the elderly and health promotion (Hughes 1993). The former were a considerable success: driving up rates due to graduated fees schedules related to the percentage of the eligible list covered. This success was repeated in 2000 when fees were introduced for influenza vaccination of the elderly and rates rose from 30 to over 80% of the eligible population. However, the other fees introduced in 1990 (e.g the annual health screening of over 75-year-olds, chronic disease management and GP-based minor surgery) remain largely evidence-free in terms of their effectiveness, let alone cost-effectiveness. This emphasizes again the need to use fees for service only to target activity at interventions of demonstrable cost-effectiveness (Scott & Maynard 1991).

The twin problems of retention and recruitment to primary care and the discontent with the independent contractor contract, particularly amongst new entrants to the profession, led to the introduction of the optional Personal Medical Service (PMS) contract in 1997, which pays GPs by salary. Unlike the 1990 reform of the contract, this new contractual option was introduced to help recruitment, retention and job flexibility, rather than to improve the performance of GPs in particular ways.

As well as PMS contracts, the government also allowed independent contractor GPs to employ other GPs directly in the same way as nurses and other practice staff. The most radical element of these reforms was that GPs could be employed by the practice thereby changing the individual contract status monopoly, which had existed since 1948.

The PMS pilots have expanded rapidly and about 20% of GPs are now contracted by salary in England. However the precise nature of these contracts and the ways in which performance has been affected and is being policed is unclear. Although salaried contracts may be regarded as having few explicit incentives for effort, implicit incentives will exist as a result of a more clear career structure (see Chapter 5). Little change in activity may be expected since the national contract is a blended payment system, and GPs may not change their activities very much when moving to salaried payment. The details of the contracts and the determination of the remuneration packages are, however, less than transparent. One national evaluation found that salaried GPs reduced the time they spent on administration and in providing out-of-hours care, although activity rates and quality of care were similar to standard contract GPs (Gosden 2002).

This result is unsurprising perhaps because socially desired behaviours are not the product of financial incentives alone. Given the complex nature of policy objectives, their pursuit requires non-price incentives as complements to payment mechanisms. These regulation and educational-based interventions include pharmaceutical prescribing feedback devices (Mason *et al.* 2001), National Institute for Clinical Excellence (NICE) recommendations, referral and practice guidelines, together with the effects, if any, of Royal College guidance and continuing medical education. Furthermore the organizational context in which activity takes place, together with the associated rules and regulations, explicit and implicit (e.g. the sense of professional duty derived from Hippocrates) is important. The effects of such incentives on the volume and quality of services delivered to patients are poorly researched. This has not, of course, inhibited policy-makers from altering remuneration contracts with little evaluation of their effects.

Robinson concludes that policy-makers involved in the reform of doctor remuneration systems would be wise to 'adopt a stance of intellectual humility and a tone of cautious optimism . . . as matters are never as good as we might hope but never as bad as we might fear' (Robinson 2001, p. 174). Such a stance would be wise given the lack of empirical work on the effects of work incentives in the public sector (Burgess & Metcalf 1999). Prendergast has also emphasized the deficiencies in the empirical evidence on work incentives on people whose work is hard to measure (e.g. GPs and their staff) and whose rewards are determined by their superiors (Prendergast 1999). Furthermore Scott has shown there is little empirical evidence about the economic consequences of the organizational structure and incentives in UK general practice (Scott 2000).

However it is unlikely that recognition of the paucity of the evidence will inform the 2002 reforms of the GP contract. The architects of these new mechanisms wish to recognize and reward the diversity of the GP's workload, improve practice infrastructure and link rewards to quality and outcome standards. These laudable aims are very similar to those that led to the reform in 1990 and remain as difficult to achieve. The salaried option will become more widely available to GPs, with those who wish to retain independent contractor status being able to do so. All GPs will provide 'essential clinical services', which will be agreed and priced nationally. 'Additional clinical services' are similar, except that practices can opt out if necessary with agreement from the local primary care organization. 'Enhanced clinical services' are where practices can 'opt in' and introduces an element of local discretion in provision and commissioning. A much larger part of GPs' income will be linked to a graded scheme of financial incentives linked to the achievement of quality standards in a number of disease areas. However, monitoring will be limited and based on principles of 'high trust and low bureaucracy' (General Practice Committee 2002).

The aims concerning improvement in quality and outcome are ambitious. The first point is one of semantics: what is meant by quality? Most patients would associate quality with improved health status, both in terms of duration of survival and functional status, as measured by health-related measures such as SF36 (www.sf36.com) and EQ5D (the Euro-QoL www.euroqol.org). Whilst the latter have been used by some practices to monitor patients' health, this has been small scale and there is no national system of quality measures in UK primary care (Williams 1997).

Such problems can only be mitigated by investment and time. In the interim it is likely that an array of imperfect process measures will be proposed as quality measures in the new contract. GPs are likely to react to these explicit incentives, but it is unclear which beneficial activities they will give up or alter to meet these targets, and whether the resulting mix of activities is efficient. 30 to 50% of income may be related to 'quality' payments related to chronic disease management. But these quality payments have no ceiling and may be inflationary and, if set poorly, inefficient. The settlement has many hidden and unevaluated costs and benefits (Marshall & Rowland 2002).

It is clear that like the PMS, the new contracting arrangements will be practice rather than individual-based. This will increase the potential for workforce substitution and might make possible actual substitution by, for instance, increasing list sizes. However the problem of data to inform performance management will remain. There are two useful sources of data, which are imperfectly exploited in primary care: hospital referral and pharmaceutical prescribing information. The drive towards electronic prescribing combined with the accumulated data held about the prescribing patterns of individual practitioners by the Prescription Pricing Authority makes it possible in principle to, for instance, monitor compliance with NICE guidelines. The system needs patient identifiers so that utilization can be linked over time and ICD diagnostic codes so that the appropriateness of prescribing can be investigated (Maynard 1998). However the PPA's capacity to store, process, record and link data over time would have to be increased by additional investment, which the Treasury has been unwilling to fund. Some GPs lament that assigning diagnostic codes is difficult, as they often do not know what is wrong with patients. However over 70% of patient contacts result in GPs prescribing something and so there appears to be some scope for improved management of pharmaceutical practice.

Another aspect of performance management that could be developed is the use of existing data collection on referrals. The Hospital Episode Statistics (HES) in England record not only details of the referring practice and practitioner but also the postcode of the patients. The former could be used to compute referral rates and the data accuracy, often questioned, would no doubt increase if this affected GP remuneration. The postcode data could be used with prescribing data to illuminate local epidemiology, as well as to show the variations by social class in the use of these NHS services.

Inherent in much of these changes is reliance on the effectiveness of performance-related pay and the virtues of team working. Again the evidence base does not support this policy optimism (see Chapter 5). Ratto and colleagues concluded 'the NHS plan welcomes the use of team rewards but neither specifies how team based incentives are to be implemented nor makes it clear to what type of teams such incentives are to be given' (Ratto *et al.* 2001, 2002). Team-related payments may work with small teams but incentives have to be complemented with the monitoring of an individual's actions and this may be complex and costly. However many of the effects of alternative team arrangements are unknown and piloting and evaluation is essential. The Department of Health's evaluation of teams is methodologically flawed and the fear must be that the 'evidence' produced will confuse rather than inform policy-making.

DEMAND-SIDE ISSUES

Access to primary care varies considerably and reflects not only differences in the supply of care locally but also variations in clinical practice, both in terms of what is delivered and the hours of opening of facilities. 'Surgery' or office hours often continue to reflect the convenience of the provider (nine to five) rather than those of the customer who wants access before and after work, and at weekends. To some extent GP co-operatives and other 'locum' mechanisms have been devised to meet these 'out-of-hours' demands and these can generate considerable sources of income for practitioners.

Quicker and more convenient access to NHS services has been central to recent policy in primary care. The centralization of GP out-of-hours provision in 1995 has provided more efficient telephone call handling. The introduction of NHS Direct and NHS Net, as well as NHS 'walk in centres', an expanding role for community pharmacists and the NHS Plan commitment to an appointment with a GP within 48 hours are all aimed at improving access to primary care. Although the effects of these initiatives on access and demand have yet to be evaluated, they raise important issues about the nature of demand. Though the GP has traditionally been the only 'gatekeeper' to the system, these new initiatives add a new set of gatekeepers. However, there is little evidence about how these new initiatives are influencing the demand for health care. Presumably, they reduce the costs of seeking advice as well as acting as a more efficient system of triage. However, this may also increase the propensity of potential patients to call with minor ailments that would otherwise have remained unknown to the health sector. Evidence suggests that NHS Direct did not act as a substitute for accident and emergency services, although it may have reduced the growth in contacts with GP out-of-hours services (Munro et al. 2000).

There is also a trade-off between more rapid access and the alleged but unproven benefits of continuity of care, traditionally a defining element of high-quality general practice. The new access initiatives suggest that rapid access is valued more highly than continuity of care by policy-makers, although there is no evidence that patients agree with this or that efficiency or equity are improved.

Geographical inequalities in the distribution of GPs have been examined and largely ignored for decades (e.g. Birch & Maynard 1986; Gravelle & Sutton 2001), even though they affect local access and, in areas of deprivation, lead to higher levels of hospital activity. Until recently, with the introduction of the PMS contract, the principal contractual policy of government was to apply 'negative direction' i.e. it declared areas 'closed' to the entry of new GPs and since 1990 offered some financial incentives (related to Jarman indices of local deprivation). Geographical funding of primary care was predominantly based on where GPs were located rather than the needs of the population. The 2002 contractual changes will facilitate the construction and application of a needs-based resource allocation formula to the whole of the primary care budget. This will direct funding to areas which have the greatest health need but which do not necessarily have the greatest capacity to produce health gains from increased investments. Such a formula is likely to be related to health and potential health gain.

The contractual approaches to improving access have had little substantive impact and as a consequence governments have adopted a more radical policy.

Perhaps the most remarkable and almost unnoticed reform of primary care in the last decade has been the increased use of nurses and other practice staff detailed earlier and, with this, many contacts with primary care are now managed by staff other than medical practitioners. This policy of de-medicalization of care has been developed further, and outside the control of GPs, by the introduction of NHS Direct and NHS 'walk in clinics'. These facilities are staffed by nurses working to simple protocols and offer much better access to advice and care. NHS Direct is a 24-hour a day telephone service and walk in clinics generally have long opening hours (particularly at the weekend and in the evenings). Neither service has been rigorously evaluated and the cautious results of the evaluation of NHS Direct pilots were largely ignored when the government 'rolled out' the service to the whole country (Munro *et al.* 1999). Ongoing evaluation of these programmes is hampered by design limitations that preclude randomized trials and with 'before and after' designs confronting the problem of bias due to anticipatory behaviour 'before' observations.

Whilst the efficiency of such innovation is unknown, its plausible effect is that access to care has been improved. No doubt the new GP contract will seek to improve access still further. Given the large increases in NHS investment by government, it is imperative that these changes be evaluated with care.

USER CHARGES FOR GP SERVICES

Despite these access improvements, the role of user charges remains an issue both in the debate about the funding of health care and the management of demand. The current government has rejected the use of user charges. However it has also 'rejected' the use of social insurance whilst at the same time introducing a flat rate (1%) national insurance increase, which in the absence of an earnings ceiling is a proportional tax identical to that used to fund social insurance schemes in mainland Europe.

Multiple methods of funding the NHS, in particular private insurance and increased user charges, are still advocated. The redistributive impact of private insurance is difficult to determine in the absence of details about tax breaks and the rules, if any, of opting out of the NHS (e.g. would such affluent leavers take with them an NHS tax credit to invest in private insurance). The attempts in Australia to increase the size of the private insurance sector by tax breaks and other policies are noticeable by the lack of evidence of their effects on efficiency and equity (Hall *et al.* 1999; Maynard & Dixon 2002).

The policy of user charges has been advocated at regular intervals for decades. Thus in 1970 the British Medical Association report on the 'failings' of the NHS argued in favour of this funding mechanism (BMA 1970). In 1995 the Health Care 2000 group, funded by the pharmaceutical industry and chaired by the former chief executive of the NHS, argued that the service was 'under funded' and that user charges were the appropriate additional funding mechanism.

What is the purpose of such advocacy? What would be the impact on access to and use of primary care? The usual arguments favouring user charges mention 'waste' and the additional funding imperative. In primary care the initial decision to consume health care is the patient's, but it is the GP that determines many of the resultant costs. The evidence shows that most patients consult a GP because they feel ill. It may be the case that an illness may be psychosomatic, e.g. the product of loneliness amongst the old. However whilst the doctors may be able to do little, the patient is in need. User charges may dissuade the needy from consulting and delays in the treatment of significant illnesses may impose higher costs on the health care system.

Canadian researchers have analysed the user charges issue at length (e.g. Stoddart *et al.* 1994). Their work illustrates the ubiquitous nature of the advocacy of these devices internationally. Further they have noted that the policy is forever being discredited but 'like a zombie', always springs back to life. Their conclusion is that this zombie-like quality is a product of pressure groups seeking to fragment the 'single pipe' tax funding (and so induce expenditure inflation and higher incomes for groups like doctors and the drug industry) and to redistribute the burden of funding health care away from richer groups in society (Evans *et al.* 1994). Unfortunately the advocates of user charges rarely make clear their redistributive goals.

In their review of the evidence of the effects of user charges Stoddart *et al.* (1994) concluded: 'most proposals for patient participation in health care financing reduce to misguided or cynical efforts to tax the ill and/or drive up the total cost of health care whilst shifting some of the burden out of government budgets'. Despite the evidence and the conclusions of these Canadian and other researchers, the user charge zombie lives on.

CONCLUSIONS

This chapter has examined a number of economic issues that are important in primary care, illustrated using examples from developments in the UK NHS. The key objective is to ensure the provision of cost-effective primary care by a motivated, productive and accountable workforce. However, there is a paucity of data and evidence in the primary care sector. Combined with the relentless and largely unevaluated reform of many aspects of primary care in the UK, the unwillingness to ensure that systems of continuous and routine data collection are in place is surprising. Managers, both clinical and non-clinical, generally ignore even the few data that are available. The new GP contract may offer an opportunity to exploit existing and develop other administrative data.

However progress will be dependent on investing in the development of the skill base (particularly the quantitative skills of managers) as well as the IT systems.

Further research is required in most areas. Recruitment and other workforce issues dominate. Little is known about the factors that influence the choice of general practice as a career, and research into the impact of the new 2002 contract on recruitment, retention and performance is essential. The role of nurses in primary care was strengthened through the 1990 GP contract, which saw the number of practice nurses double to deliver the contract's commitments. However, lack of data has prevented a systematic analysis of the effects of changes to skill mix. This could be achieved through the estimation of cost functions, which could indicate whether the nurses are substitutes or complements for GPs. There is also a lack of data on the role of the wider primary care team, hence this chapter's inevitable focus on GPs. The new 2002 contract may reduce the previous barriers to changing skill mix, and careful evaluation is required.

The advent of increased consumer choice at the point of access to the NHS also merits further research, particularly in terms of the level of demand and equality of access. It is also essential to determine whether the resources being invested in these initiatives could have been better spent elsewhere.

Policy-making continues to be based on the principle of designing and implementing change on the basis of 'by guess and by God'. Many recent policies, such as NHS Direct, walk in centres and advocacy of performance-related pay are ill defined and poorly costed. Limited evaluation has taken place, and this has served merely to wrap policy in the myth of evaluation whilst failing to produce robust 'evidence' of the consequences of reform.

Primary care remains a 'black box' where the processes, let alone the outcomes of care, are poorly described let alone evaluated. The government is now embarking on another period of reform and has promised a major and ambitious increase in the funding of the system. As Campbell remarked over 30 years ago all such reform is a social experiment which can and should be evaluated to ensure the knowledge base grows systematically (Campbell 1969). For the last 35 years this advocacy of a scientific approach to policy design and implementation has been ignored, with politicians preferring to operate behind what Campbell called the 'veil of ignorance'. It is to be regretted that such 'traditions' of policy-making die hard.

ACKNOWLEDGEMENTS

We would like to thank Nick Bosanquet and participants of the HERU workshop for helpful comments. HERU is funded by the Chief Scientist Office of the Scottish Executive Health Department. The views are those of the authors.

REFERENCES

Birch S and Maynard A (1986) *The RAWP review, rawping primary care and rawping the United Kingdom.* Discussion Paper 19, Centre for Health Economics, University of York.

Bloor K and Maynard A (2001) Workforce productivity and incentive structures in the UK National Health Service. *Journal of Health Service Research and Policy*, **6**(2), 105–113.

Bloor K, Maynard A and Street A (2000) The cornerstone of Labour's New NHS: reforming primary care. In Smith PC (Ed.), *Reforming Markets in Health Care.* Open University Press, Buckingham.

BMA (British Medical Association) (1970) *Health Services Financing*, London.

Burgess S and Metcalfe P (1999) *Incentives in organisations: a selective overview of the literature with application to the public sector.* Centre for Market and Public Organisation, Working Paper No. 99/016, University of Bristol.

Campbell DT (1969) Reforms as experiments. *American Psychologist*, **24**(4), 409–429.

Cooper RA, Laud P and Dietrich CL (1998) Current and projected workforce of nonphysician clinicians. *Journal of the American Medical Association*, **280**, 788–794.

Department of Social Security (1986) *Primary health care: an agenda for discussion.* HMSO, London.

Elliott RF, Mavromaras K, Scott A, Bell DNF, Antonazzo E, Gerova V and Van der Pol M (2002) *Labour markets and NHS Scotland.* Report to Scottish Executive Health Department, University of Aberdeen.

Evans RG, Barer ML, Stoddart G and Bhatia V (1994) *Who are the Zombie masters and what do they want?* Premier's Council on Health, Well-being and Social Justice, Ottawa.

General Practice Committee (2002) *Your contract, your future.* British Medical Association, London.

Gosden T (2002) *Paying doctors by salary: the influence on GP behaviour in Personal Medical Services (PMS) pilot sites in England.* PhD Thesis, University of Manchester.

Gosden T, Bowler I and Sutton M (2000) How do general practitioners choose their practice? Preferences for practice and job characteristics. *Journal of Health Services Research and Policy*, **5**, 208–213.

Gosden T, Forland F, Kristiansen IS, Sutton M, Leese B, Guiffrida A, Sergison M and Pedersen L (2001) Impact of payment method on the behaviour of primary care physicians: a systematic review. *Journal of Health Services Research and Policy*, **6**, 44–55.

Gravelle H and Sutton M (2001) Inequalities in the geographical distribution of GPs in England and Wales 1974–1995. *Journal of Health Services Research and Policy*, **6**, 6–13.

Hall J, De Abreu Lourenco R and Viney R (1999) Carrots and sticks: the fall and fall of private health insurance in Australia. *Health Economics*, **8**(8), 653–660.

Harris Interactive (2002) *Health Care News*, **2**, 13.

Health Care (2000) *UK Health and Health Care Services: challenges and policy options.* Glaxo, 1995.

HM Treasury (2002). *Opportunity and security for all: investing in an enterprising fairer Britain.* New Public Spending Plans, 2003–2006. HM Treasury, London.

Horrocks S, Anderson E and Salisbury C (2002) Systematic review of whether nurse practitioners working in primary care can provide equivalent care to doctors. *British Medical Journal,* **324**, 819–823.

Horton R (2002) Nurse prescribing in the UK: right but also wrong. *Lancet* (editorial) **359**, 9321.

Hughes D (1993) General practitioners and the new contract: promoting better health through financial incentives. *Health Policy,* **25**, 39–50.

Marshall M and Roland M (2002) The new contract: renaissance or requiem for general practice. *British Journal of General Practice,* **52**, 1.

Mason J, Freemantle N, Narareth I, Eccles M, Haines A and Drummond M (2001) When is it cost effective to change the behavior of health professionals? *Journal of the American Medical Association,* **286**, 2988–2992.

Maynard A (1998) Who should control GP prescribing? *Update,* p. 565.

Maynard A and Dixon A (2002) Private insurance and medical savings accounts: theory and practice. In E Mossialos, A Dixon *et al.* (Eds), *Funding Health Care: Options for Europe.* Open University Press, Buckingham.

Maynard A and Dowson S (1985) *Health Care.* King's Fund, London.

Mundinger MO, Kane RL, Lenz ER *et al.* (2000) Primary care outcomes in patients treated by nurse practitioners or physicians. *Journal of the American Medical Association,* **283**, 59–68.

Munro J, Nicholl J, O'Cathain A and Knowles E (1999) *Evaluation of NHS Direct first wave sites.* First Interim Report to the Department of Health. Medical Care Research Unit, University of Sheffield.

Munro J, Nicholl J, O'Caithain A and Knowles E (2000) Impact of NHS Direct on demand for immediate care: observational study. *British Medical Journal,* **321**, 150–153.

Office of Health Economics (2000) *Compendium of Health Statistics,* 12th Edition, London.

Prendergast C (1999) The provision of incentives in firms. *Journal of Economic Literature,* **37**, 7–63.

Ratto M, Burgess S, Croxson B, Jewitt I and Propper C (2001) *Team-based incentives in the NHS; an economic analysis,* Centre for Market and Public Organisation, Working Paper No. 01/37, University of Bristol.

Ratto M, Propper C and Burgess S (2002) Using financial incentives to promote teamwork in health care. *Journal of Health Services Research and Policy,* 7(2), 69–70.

Richardson, Maynard A, Cullum N and Kindig D (1998) Skill mix changes: substitution or service development? *Health Policy,* **45**, 119–132.

Robinson JC (2001) Theory and practice in the design of physician payment incentives. *Milbank Memorial Fund Quarterly,* **79**(2), 149–177.

Scott A (2000) Economics of general practice. In AJ Culyer and JP Newhouse (Eds), *Handbook of Health Economics.* Elsevier, Amsterdam.

Scott A (2001) Eliciting GPs' preferences for pecuniary and non-pecuniary job characteristics. *Journal of Health Economics,* **20**, 329–347.

Scott A and Maynard A (1991) *Will the new GP contract lead to cost effective medical practice?* Discussion Paper 82, Centre for Health Economics, University of York.

Seddon ME, Marshall MN, Campbell SM and Roland MO (2001) Systematic review of studies of quality of clinical care in general practice in the UK, Australia and New Zealand. *Quality in Health Care,* **10**, 152–158.

Sibbald B, Bojke C and Gravelle H (2002) National survey of job satisfaction and retirement intentions among general practitioners in England. *British Medical Journal* (forthcoming).

Sox HC (2000) Independent primary care by nurse practitioners. *Journal of the American Medical Association*, **283**(1) (editorial).

Starfield B (1998) *Primary Care: Balancing Health Needs, Services and Technology*. Oxford University Press, Oxford.

Stoddart GL, Barer ML and Evans RG (1994) *User Charges, Snares and Delusions: another look at the literature*. Premier's Council on Health, Well-being and Social Justice, Ontario.

Weiner JP (1991) Forecasting the effects of health reform on US physicians workforce requirements. *Journal of the American Medical Association*, **272**, 220–230.

Wilkin D and Metcalf DHM (1984) List size and patient contact in general practice. *British Medical Journal*, **289**, 1501–1505.

Williams A (1997) The measurement and valuation of health: a chronicle. In AJ Culyer and A Maynard (Eds), *Being Reasonable About the Economics of Health: selected essays by Alan Williams*. Edward Edgar, Cheltenham.

11

Equity in Health Care: The Need for a New Economics Paradigm?

GAVIN MOONEY
Social and Public Health Economics Research Group (SPHERe), Curtin University,
Perth

ELIZABETH RUSSELL
Department of Public Health, University of Aberdeen

INTRODUCTION

In the public sector economists traditionally have attempted to work with a social welfare function that is frequently based on some simple aggregation of individual preferences. This is in essence a welfarist basis where it is assumed not only that it is the preferences of individuals *qua* individuals, manifested through choice, which are to count but also that each individual is attempting to maximize his or her own welfare or utility. The idea that individuals might be interested to contribute to some common good which at the same time might result in a lowering of their own utility is not permitted. This 'counterpreferential' concept, built into for example commitment, is, as Sen (1977) indicates, not present in welfarism. Also absent, since welfarism is consequentialist, is any argument in the welfare function which is represented by process where the process is valued in itself and not just as instrumental towards some outcome.

In an attempt to overcome some of the problems of welfarism in health care, Culyer (1990) introduced the paradigm of 'extra welfarism' into health economics which, *inter alia*, shifted the contents of the objective function from utility to health. He suggested that this shift is based on some 'external judgement' but he does not go on to explain from where this external judgement came. In the specific context of equity, that may leave some problems in its

Advances in Health Economics. Edited by Anthony Scott, Alan Maynard and Robert Elliott.
© 2003 John Wiley & Sons, Ltd

wake, not least being the questions of (a) whether health maximization is the goal of health care and (b) who should determine what that goal should be.

There has been considerable effort expended by several health economists over the years to examining various facets of equity in health care (see for example Mooney 1987; Culyer 1990; Wagstaff & van Doorslaer 1992; Donaldson & Gerard 1993; Mooney 1996; Williams 1997; McIntyre & Gilson 2000; Wiseman & Jan 2000). Their contributions have been to the understanding and analysis of equity in health care. This chapter takes a rather different look at equity and suggests *inter alia* that a new paradigm may now be more relevant to how equity is perceived and analysed in the 21st century.

It is argued that both welfarism and extra welfarism (as normally construed) suffer from what are identified as two major problems in addressing equity: first each takes account only of individuals' values and not community values and second each assumes that all that is in the objective function is both measurable and commensurable (utility in the case of welfarism and health in extra welfarism). It would seem to require only one of these characteristics to create some problems for current health economics approaches to equity. It is also the case that while the blame cannot be laid solely at the door of health economists, policies in health care have, by and large and across the globe, failed to deliver equity in the last 20 to 30 years. The chapter concludes more positively with an alternative approach which still needs to be worked out in detail but which may offer a better road to address equity in health care. This is based partly on the work of Sen (1992) but also draws on communitarianism and the concept of 'communitarian claims'.

In essence this alternative starts from the premise that communities as well as individuals have values and that these community values may be different from the aggregate of individual values. It is argued first that it is not the values of individuals *qua* individuals which should be used as the preference base in addressing equity, but rather the values of the community that these individuals comprise; second that there are problems in adopting a single set of preferences across different social groupings, for example different cultures; third that the preferences of those deemed to be being treated inequitably should be the basis for the allocation of any resources they receive to address their inequities; fourth that the ability to 'manage to desire' is unlikely to be constant across all groups in society (Sen 1992) and in particular may well be truncated or muffled in those currently being treated inequitably; and finally that the obsession with measurement and quantification can lead economics down an unhelpful reductionist road.

The belief that community values exist mirrors the recognition that Adam Smith (1759) gave to the need for rules, essentially social or community rules. Smith wrote: 'without regard to ... general rules ... what would become of the duties of justice, of truth, of chastity, of fidelity ...? ... upon the tolerable observance of these duties, depends the very existence of human society, which would crumble into nothing if mankind were not generally impressed with a reverence for those important rules of conduct.'

The reason for quoting Smith is that this amounts to a criticism of what today would be deemed a welfarist perspective. Again if welfarists want to argue that justice, truth, chastity and fidelity can all be built into welfarism, then it would begin to appear as if there is nothing that is not welfarism. Any conception of extra welfarism or non-welfarism would then be redundant. Any categorization however that allows everything to be in a single category is not worthy of the term 'categorization'. This is relevant because welfarists sometimes create an impression that nothing is or could be beyond welfarism.

There is a large literature in economics under the heading of public choice and social choice theory that might have been built into this chapter (see for example Buchanan & Mathieu 1986; Mueller 1989; Schokkaert 1992). That literature suggests other ways of dealing with the issues here but is not directly relevant to the arguments presented here because it does not address an explicit communitarian approach, which is what is seen as fundamental in the paradigm set out below.

In the next section welfarism and Sen's critique of welfarism (see for example Sen 1992) is outlined, followed by a description and then a critique of extra welfarism in the third and fourth sections. How to move forward with equity in health care is set out in the fifth section, followed by a brief conclusion in the final section.

WELFARISM AND SEN'S CRITIQUE

Welfarism can take different guises. It is not the intent here to attempt to argue that it is not in some contexts useful. Here the concern is with equity and there are seeming limitations of the welfarist approach in how it handles equity. Fundamentally with respect to welfare, it is normally argued that any welfare is derived by individuals as individuals and that such welfare is derived only from goods or commodities. Value is obtained from welfare which in turn is seen as involving pleasure, happiness or desire (Sen 1992). There are a number of different ways in which welfarism tackles the issue of aggregation to some social welfare function, most simply for example by adding together individuals' welfares. Welfarism also usually assumes that individuals seek to maximize their own individual welfare.

Sen is critical of such welfarism (Sen 1992). Crucial in Sen's approach are what he calls 'functionings' and 'capabilities' (Sen 1985). Sen wants to go beyond commodities, in the conventional welfare economics sense. He recognizes that individuals are different in terms of their abilities to convert commodities into ways of providing themselves with well-being so that, even if goods were allocated equally across different individuals, this would not necessarily lead to equal well-being or utility. An individual's functionings are 'what he or she manages to do or to be' (Sen 1985, p. 10). 'Capabilities' are about freedoms or opportunities to choose. Thus capabilities represent the freedoms that an individual has in terms of the range of functionings that the individual faces by way of choice. Functionings are what are achieved from some range of capabilities; they are realized capabilities. It is also not assumed by Sen that the individual will necessarily choose to maximize her own well-being as he allows for other possible motives for choice (such as obligations to others).

Sen is particularly keen to distinguish between his concepts of well-being and advantage on the one hand and utility on the other. He suggests there is a need to allow for 'a variety of human acts and states as important in themselves (not just because they may produce utility, nor just to the extent that they yield utility)' (Sen 1985, p. 22). His concerns with respect to the narrowness of utilitarianism are particularly strong at the level of interpersonal variations and comparisons.

Sen (1985) argues that the utility tradition suffers from two problems: that of what he calls 'physical-condition neglect' and that of 'valuation neglect'. A person who suffers from physical condition neglect (for example he is undernourished) 'can still be high up in the scale of happiness or desire-fulfilment if he or she has learned to have "realistic" desires and to take pleasure in small mercies' (Sen 1985, p. 23). Further he claims, with respect to valuation neglect: 'Valuing is not the same thing as desiring, and the strength of desire is influenced by considerations of realism in one's circumstances.' Sen further argues (Sen 1992, p. 149) that 'an overdependence on what people "manage to desire" is one of the limiting aspects of utilitarian ethics, which is particularly neglectful of the claims of those who are too subdued or broken to have the courage to desire much.' This is perhaps Sen's most telling criticism of welfarism and is a crucially important point in assessing equity and a large part of why this chapter calls for a new paradigm.

The source of valuing that Sen uses remains, as with welfarism, with the individual (although when Sen raises the question of certain individuals' inability to 'manage to desire' the source of values becomes less clear). Sen is particularly scathing of those who would not allow variations in individuals' values. Thus he writes (Sen 1992, p. 30): 'The tendency to assume away interpersonal diversities [of values] can originate not only from the pragmatic temptation to make the analytics simple and easy (*as in the literature of inequality measurement*), but also ... from the rhetoric of equality itself (e.g. "all men are created equal").' (Emphasis added.)

Finally, Sen argues strongly on two issues related to measurement. He suggests first (Sen 1993) that the purpose of the evaluation will and should influence what is in the evaluative space, i.e. what is to be measured. Second, he suggests that measurement can be taken too far and he seeks to guard against 'over' completeness. '"Waiting for toto" may not be a cunning strategy in a practical exercise' (Sen 1992, p. 49). He argues that (Sen 1992, p. 48) 'the nature of interpersonal comparisons of well-being...as a discipline may admit incompleteness as a regular part of the...exercise...An approach that can rank the well-being of every person against that of every other in a straightforward way...may well be at odds with the nature of these ideas.'

There is thus a very real difference between Sen's position and the utilitarian stance. If analysts however are not to rely on what people 'manage to desire', then how are they to find out what people would desire if they did get round to managing?

This is an important issue. It is central to the question of equity in health care. For example, if some people do not manage to desire good health, should that position be respected by health care policy-makers or should it somehow be adjusted to 'compensate for the inadequate' values that emerge from such individuals? If other people do not manage to desire good health enough or if yet others are prepared to settle for a rather lower level of health than some do, or that others would if they were in the same circumstances, then what?

This anti-welfarist stance by Sen manifests itself in another but related way. He expresses concern that individuals may be deprived and as a result their desires constrained. He writes (Sen 1985, p. 29): 'A poor, undernourished person, brought up in penury, may have learned to come to terms with a half-empty stomach, seizing joy in small comforts and desiring no more than what seems "realistic".' And he adds immediately: 'But this mental attitude does not wipe out the fact of the person's deprivation.' That in turn raises questions regarding who is to define the level below which, and of what, people are deemed to be 'deprived' and hence whose desires are not 'realistic'.

EXTRA WELFARISM

DESCRIPTION OF EXTRA WELFARISM

Some detail on extra welfarism is relevant to this chapter, especially as spelt out by Culyer in his normative economics paper of 1990, which was the first specific reference to this paradigm within health economics (Culyer 1990). Some comments are set out here from Culyer's original work to explain some of the content of extra welfarism before then mounting a critique.

Culyer (1990) argued that in welfarism the only source of welfare or utility is goods and services and that leaves out some other potentially important aspects of individuals such as their ability to choose. He then proposed that extra welfarism allows other features of individuals to be included. Thus, whereas welfarism traditionally encompasses only goods, Culyer's extra welfarism in principle opens the door to any and all *non-goods* based utility, but still focuses on individuals.

Particularly important to Culyer's (1990) position is that there is scope in extra welfarism for some external judgement being applied as to what is to count and what is not to count. This directly contradicts the welfarist view that it is only individual preferences that are to count. Culyer went on to argue that health is identified by extra welfarists as the principal output of health care services.

With respect to measurement issues in extra welfarism, it is normally assumed that the contents of the objective function, i.e. health, are measurable (usually through QALYs). Further, it is assumed that individual preferences count but that beyond that individuals' preferences for own health are not allowed to influence the value attached to their own health gains compared with others' health gains. Culyer also suggests that his extra welfarism is heavily dependent on Sen's critique of welfarism.

CRITIQUE OF EXTRA WELFARISM

Some of the criticisms of extra welfarism also apply to welfarism. Thus the notion that all that is in the objective function can be quantified is an assumption which welfarism and extra welfarism share and which Sen opposes. In the context of equity, it is shown below that this is a crucial argument from Sen.

Turning now to criticisms which are specific to extra welfarism, certainly any move to endorsing the notion that non-goods utilities or interests are to be included is desirable and allows *inter alia* for the inclusion of process for which GM (see for example Mooney 1994) has been arguing for some time. However Culyer's claim that extra welfarism relies heavily on Sen is disputed. As indicated, Sen himself makes very clear with respect to his central concept of capabilities that he is opposed to the utilitarian calculus. Sen is not extra welfarist; he is *non*-welfarist.

Certainly Culyer's extra welfarism and Sen's critique of welfarism share a view of the world that there are aspects of each social state other than simply goods and services which are relevantly included in the evaluation space. Yet in the remainder of the paper in which he makes the point, and in papers since, Culyer has restricted the focus solely to *health*.

In practical terms therefore the way that Culyer uses 'extra welfarism' is rather limited. He shifts the contents of the evaluative space from goods to health. Given, as demonstrated in the previous section, how Sen attempts to encompass so much within his concept of a person's interests, it seems likely that he would go far beyond this view if he were to address the same issue.

If a fuller view is taken of Sen's critique of welfarism, the issue of health as the maximand becomes a red herring. Nowhere is there any sense in which Sen treats health as synonymous with 'capabilities'. Culyer did health economics a favour in moving the subdiscipline further away from welfarism, but his suggestion even tentatively that all that there is in the objective function is health has not been as useful.

There is thus an argument for endorsing the idea of there being external judgements which are used to decide what the objective function of health care is to be. It is important however to pin down, as attempted in the next section, the source of these external judgements and not leave them, as Culyer seems to do, *ex cathedra*.

Two external judgements are built into extra welfarism. One, health maximization, has already been discussed. The second is the view that variations in individuals' valuations of own health should not be allowed. Certainly in their ignorance of what is wrong with them, of what treatments are available and of their likely effectiveness, individuals are often deficient in being able to make rational choices with respect to health care consumption. That does not mean necessarily that there is something wrong with their preferences or at least nothing more wrong with their preferences for *health* than with their preferences for other facets of their lives – how they value freedom, their preferences for education, their preferences for law and order, etc. If certain individuals, on an informed and rational basis but one which could not be classified as deprived (see section 2), value their health more highly or conversely more lowly than others, it might be that the objective function for health care should reflect this. The idea within extra welfarism that an external judgement should be made that such variations are not to be allowed is, as a minimum, in need of defence. Culyer does not offer one. The idea that there might be an external judgement about such matters is not something that should necessarily be questioned. There is an argument however for having the content of such external judgements justified or legitimized in some way or other. The justification from Smith and from the authors is that there is a community dimension to preferences and values that in some circumstances may over-ride those of the individual: equity may be one such circumstance.

There *is* something to be said for Culyer's extra welfarism. It must be apparent however that the assumption that health is the only argument in the objective function of health care is only one of many possible assumptions that might be defined as extra welfarist.

Thus there appear to be various conceptual and ethical problem areas in both welfarism and extra welfarism. First, each remains firmly in a world where individual preferences determine the values or weights to be attached to whatever states are to be considered. Second, they are consequentialist (indeed very narrowly consequentialist in extra welfarism when the only outcome in the objective function is health). Third, they do not allow for differential relevance of valuations or preferences in different contexts. In respect of equity, the stance adopted in this chapter (and recognizing there is no ethically neutral position on this) is that it is a principle of equity that the preferences of the disadvantaged should be reflected in how health care resources are used to assist disadvantaged groups. (In Australia for example it is increasingly recognized that not to respect the preferences of Aboriginal people in the design and operation of health care for them is unhelpful to their self-esteem and in turn to their health. See for example Houston 2001.) It follows *inter alia* that it is then not possible to use a single system of values in applying equity policy.

The question remains how to decide what proportion of health care resources is to be allocated to different individuals or subgroups of a community defined by a particular characteristic. If all groups did have an equal capacity to manage to desire, then presumably some aggregation of each group's utilities could be used in the allocation of resources. However, there is ample evidence that the capacity to manage to desire will vary both culturally and socially (see for example Houston 2001). If different groups also have a different construct of health, then the situation becomes yet more difficult. How can the distribution of apples and oranges be equalized or even simply treated fairly when there can be no reliance on any comparison of the utilities that the two groups get from apples and oranges and indeed it is not even known in advance when the allocation is made that one group will not spend the money on pears?

A NEW PARADIGM

Given the above criticisms of both welfarism and extra welfarism, it is suggested that there is a need for an alternative that will allow society to determine how the resources for equity in health care are to be allocated.[1] This new economics paradigm for equity in health care must be able to accommodate: (i) community values at the level of choosing an equity goal and deciding on relative weights to be attached to different inequities (e.g. by socio-economic status or by geographical area); (ii) the idea that there may be value in the community *per se* and that counterpreferential choices at the individual level may not be counterpreferential at the community level; (iii) the principle that preferences of those groups treated inequitably should form the basis for how their inequities are then addressed; and (iv) the idea that

---

[1] There is of course no reason why this approach need be restricted to health care. It could be argued that all goods be handled in this way. It is likely however that for most goods the market will remain the method of choice for such allocations except where there is clear market failure as in the case of health care (personal communication, Mavromaras 2002).

the method for allocating resources equitably may not be able to use some set of measurable outcomes in deciding what is equitable. The conceptual framework adopted is based on various ideas but it comes primarily from Smith (1759) and Sen (1992). Its essence is communitarian (see for example Aveneri & de Shalit 1992). Important insights into policy-making on equity can be obtained if there is an attempt to adopt or at least to understand the communitarian perspective. Taking such a stand means that there is an interest in social values and aggregation of the preferences, interests or whatever of individuals not just *qua* individuals, but also as part of a community or society where the community itself is valued.

The fundamentals of the communitarian approach in this context are as follows. First communitarians assume that it is the community's preferences which should decide on the principles underlying the social institution which is the health care system, and the way in which these principles should be operationalized. In the context of equity this means that the concept of equity in health care and the relative weight attached to it in the health care objective function are to be determined according to community preferences. Second, such community preferences may not be the same as the aggregation of individuals' preferences. Third, the idea of establishing what may be best described as the social good of health care (perhaps, but not necessarily, through Sen's 'capabilities') is important in communitarianism. Fourth since different individuals, and more importantly at this level different groupings, within society (poor people, coloured people) may have different abilities to manage to desire adequately, which appears to be the case with respect to health for different cultural groupings (see Wiseman 1999), even if there were a desire to place all of these preferences on a single measuring rod (such as utility) it is not legitimate to do so. (As discussed earlier, this situation is even more problematical if health and/or health need are different constructs in different social groupings as they may well be for example across different cultural groups.)

To argue as is done here for this new paradigm requires establishing first that the old paradigm is in some sense flawed. The reliance on individual values in existing paradigms may be seen as a flaw although not necessarily (even if the authors are of the view that a more communitarian approach is advantageous). An inability on the part of some groups to manage to desire adequately, if accepted as the authors do, is a flaw in the welfarist approach. Not having a defence of the basis of any external judgement about what is to be contained in the objective function is problematical yet that is what extra welfarism is based upon. Where there are different constructs of health across for example different cultures, then extra welfarism cannot continue to rely on a common metric for health. The implication of much of welfarism is also exposed to doubt on this point.

The new paradigm requires that society has recognized the issues of managing to desire differentially and of pluralistic values. The latter could be coped with by aggregation. What cannot is the sense of a community having values that accept the principle of ceding importance to someone else or to some other group, i.e. the community. Further, if either of the existing economic paradigms, welfarism or extra-welfarism, had been widely accepted and used, then to propose an alternative paradigm would be less or even inappropriate. Neither has.

Communitarian claims (Mooney 1998, 2001) go a long way to overcoming these problems. They may therefore be useful in getting the community to determine how to allocate health care resources equitably across different competing groups.

Turning to communitarianism more explicitly, in the debate between that philosophy and the libertarians and individualists, the key difference lies in how society is conceived. As Taylor (1989, p. 47) writes: 'The crucial point here is this: since the free individual can only maintain his identity within a society/ culture of a certain kind, he has to be concerned about the shape of this society/ culture as a whole. He cannot . . . be concerned purely with his individual choices and the associations formed from such choices to the neglect of the matrix in which such choices can be open or closed, rich or meagre. It is important to him that certain activities and institutions flourish in society. It is even of importance to him what the moral tone of the whole society is . . . because freedom and individual diversity can only flourish in a society where there is a general recognition of their worth.' He continues: 'If realizing our freedom partly depends on the society and culture in which we live, then we exercise a fuller freedom if we can help determine the shape of this society and culture.'

While there are different routes to examine this, useful here is Sen's notion of capabilities (as discussed in section 2). These seem particularly germane in health care. QALYs as measures of health are restricted to just that and are normally constrained to valuing what people achieve in a health state. They ignore what the person's capabilities are at two levels: first, the capabilities in the state the individual is in currently; and second, the capabilities in moving to some state other than the one the individual is in. Individuals in a particular health state have certain functionings (which is where we interpret the QALY to lie) but they also have the opportunity or the freedom to choose from a range of functionings – 'capabilities' in Sen's terms (but clearly constrained by their health status). What different people are capable of in the same health state varies. Some cope better than others. Some have different objectives and consequently have different incentives to adjust to their health state. It may be useful to talk about health services seeking to do good. It is both possible and fruitful to get policy-makers and others to get into debate about the question: 'what is the good of health care?' Everyone seems able to take part in that debate and bring less baggage to it than if they continue with the language of the welfarist and extra welfarist schools.

Those in favour of communitarianism (Aveneri & de Shalit 1992) argue for the community to be centre stage. Community can be defined in different ways. For the purposes of this chapter it is simply a group of people with some common life through reciprocity, mutuality and sharing. Communitarians thus stress the social, with individuals' identities and relationships being communally based. Communitarianism can be contrasted with the atomism of modern liberalism. It is not just community spirit but a recognition, beyond that, that the community is something to be valued in and of itself. Individuals not only see themselves as members of a community but their identities are shaped by such membership. Their preferences are not independent of the community in which they act, live or work. They will be members of various communities, some of which may overlap. In the context of health care they may be members of a local community which is served by local community services; be registered with a particular general practice; fall within a particular hospital catchment area; be a citizen of Scotland. At each of these levels the 'community' is different and the interests of the community may well be different. Being in a GP practice, the preferences of the practice population will relate to the activities of the GPs and staff and revolve around issues of technical care, opening hours and accessibility more generally, etc. At a citizen level however one may be interested in much broader issues such as accessibility to health care generally for different groups as a function of, for example, what is seen as a decent society.

How to elicit community and communitarian preferences is not the subject of this chapter. These two sets of preferences are likely to be similar. The difference between them, in principle at least, lies in the emphasis that communitarians place on the embeddedness of people in communities with the resultant sharing, reciprocity and mutuality that will exist in more communitarian communities. In practice there is likely to be a continuum from more individualistic communities to more communitarian communities.

Some research has been done on eliciting community preferences: see for example Abelson and Lomas (1996) and Leneghan (1999). There is also some limited evidence that asking people as individuals and asking them as state planners gives different answers (Mooney *et al.* 1999; Jan *et al.* 2000). The latter however would still seem to fall short of what might be more genuinely community preferences. It would be advantageous in making the case for a new paradigm if it were possible to spell out first how to obtain community and communitarian preferences and second show that these differ from the aggregation of individual preferences. That cannot be done in any detail at this time. There is however research which attempts to establish community preferences using for example citizens' juries (Leneghan 1999; Medical Council 2000, 2001). There has been little evaluation of such activities and none that compares the aggregation of individualistically based preferences with community values.

There may be those who worry that if this paradigm is accepted certain groups will miss out, e.g. minority groups such as the mentally handicapped. It is difficult in advance of testing this approach empirically to know if that fear is justified. It is not in the authors' view already the case that minorities are well protected currently. Experience with citizens' juries in Australia is potentially relevant as to how minority groups might fare under the new paradigm. One jury (Medical Council 2000), drawn totally from the city of Perth, voted for a greater proportion of additional health care resources being allocated to rural and remote parts of the state rather than to Perth. Two other juries (Medical Council 2001), on whom no Aboriginal people sat, voted for high weights, reflecting positive discrimination/vertical equity in favour of Aboriginal people. Whether such protection of minorities would stand up to more general appraisal remains to be seen.

What communitarianism does is provide an alternative to welfarism and extra welfarism. Together with Virginia Wiseman, GM has previously argued for the idea of a 'constitution' as the vehicle for expressing this communitarianism (Mooney & Wiseman 2000). The notion of a 'constitution' for health services comes from what Vanberg (1994, p. 135) describes as 'the constitutional paradigm', which 'reverses . . . the logic of the goal paradigm'. Instead of concentrating on the 'goals that organizational action is supposedly *directed at*, it draws attention to the procedural foundations that organizational action is *based upon*.' One of the gaps in UK health policy-making and priority setting is any informed forum in which even the voting community can express its communal and consensus views on preferences for NHS developments and fundamentals. In Western Australia, in the South West Health Service, there are plans to hold a constitutional convention.

What might this constitution look like? It is a set of principles on which policy and actions might be based: things like equity and how important it is and how it might be defined. Is there to be concern only with horizontal equity and the equal treatment of equals or also vertical equity and the unequal but equitable treatment of unequals? It might get into issues of respect for individual autonomy and, for example, ensuring the freedom of individuals to refuse treatment. It might consider the extent to which it is only outcomes that matter or also process. For example *the process* of decision-making seems to be a matter of some importance to Aboriginal people – perhaps more so or at least more explicitly than is normally assumed for non-indigenous people. In the UK, political scientists such as Hunter (1997) and Klein (1998) advocate explicit process, rather than outcomes, as the only feasible focus for involving the public and its values in priority setting. It might even state in which contexts in public health the community's preferences should count and when they, the community, feel willing and able to leave it to the experts. Leading into this can be achieved through 'communitarian claims' (Mooney 1998). Such claims 'recognise first that the duty is owed by the community of which the candidate is a member and secondly that the carrying out of this duty is not just instrumental but is good in itself' (Mooney 1998, p. 1176).

The word 'claim' is perhaps an unfortunate one in this context as in everyday usage it tends to require an active role for the person who is to benefit from the claim. 'I claim' and 'you claim' is standard usage where this is shorthand for 'I claim on my behalf' and 'you claim on your behalf'. Here we *the community* determine how resources are allocated on the basis of how we *the community* see various different groups' or individuals' strengths of claims for the resources involved. It is *our* preferences, the community's preferences, for *their* claims, the various groups' claims, that determine how the resources are allocated. It is we *the community* who also decide what is relevant in identifying and weighting claims in terms of the characteristics of the different potential recipient groups and the community as a whole.

One aspect of this that is important to recognize – and it is argued that this is crucially important – is that these communitarian claims are not welfarist. They allow the society or the community to decide who shall have access to what quantities of resources for what purposes. They accept that resources are limited and provide a community-determined mechanism for their allocation to competing groups. They are thus about community provision. There is no need strictly for the recipients to be active in 'claiming' the resources. There is also no implied absolute right of any individual to consume any service. There cannot be any absolute right given the acceptance of scarcity. The claim establishes the legitimacy of that service for that individual (or more likely for a group into which that individual falls). The extent to which that service in practice is provided will in turn hinge on the community's judgement of the strengths of claims involved and the resources available.

The actual *consumption* of the resources however remains inevitably and rightly determined by how individuals value the options with which they are then faced. It may also be the case (as with the Margolis 1982 fair shares model) that there is a 'loop' here, such that if certain groups, in some sense or other that the community seeks to favour, do not use or misuse the resources made available to them, this may influence the community in assessing claims and strengths of claims next time round.

Over the longer term and going back to 1963 and Arrow's seminal article then about the nature of the commodity health care (Arrow 1963), economists have tended to focus more on the problems for consumers in valuing *health care*. It is only more recently that there has been the (near) obsession with valuing *health*. In judging whether variations in individuals' values for health are to count in the objective function then here is perhaps the perfect example of where the community can express its preferences. It can choose to argue that all preferences should be treated as equal or it can allow preferences to vary. It can also choose within the latter to allow variations for some reasons but not for others. Here are issues that the community might want to examine in establishing principles or a constitution for a health care system.

In practice, explicit community values and principles have already been established in a number of nations and states around the world. Two of the most widely publicized are Oregon, USA and Sweden. In Oregon, the over-riding principle was equity of access for non-insured persons in the state. They have achieved this by increasing the numbers eligible for health care through a prioritization programme that limits the use of certain clinical procedures (Garland 2001). Crucially, the priorities were chosen through an extensive public and health care consultation process that involved special effort (by no means totally successful) to obtain the views of those who were not insured as well as those who were. In Sweden, a Commission – again using extensive public and health care consultation – established a set of ethical principles that led them to agree that patients who were severely or chronically ill, or in terminal care, were being disadvantaged compared to those with acute diseases and should receive positive policy discrimination (Swedish Parliamentary Priorities Commission 1995).

In Scotland, inequality of life expectancy has been the driver for the current health strategy, which prioritizes inequality of life circumstances and life styles as targets for health resources (Scottish Executive Health Department 1998). In the UK since 1976, health service resource allocation has attempted to take account of social deprivation as reflected by mortality. The Arbuthnott formula for resource allocation to health boards within Scotland incorporates measures of 'unmet need' to reflect inequalities in local morbidity, life circumstances and rurality (Scottish Executive Health Department 1999). What is less clear is whether local activities reflect these priorities. The point for this chapter is that these political priorities have almost entirely ignored any economic paradigms, whether welfarism or extra welfarism; economics to date has been marginalized.

This new paradigm in principle allows the debate on equity to move forward. It places equity firmly in the social box and removes it from the individualistic and essentially selfish preferences that to date have driven both welfarist and extra welfarist notions of equity. In its at least implicit appeal to altruism in the setting of claims to health care resources, it allows something beyond individualistic notions of welfare, of health and of social institutions to be centre stage. It also avoids some of the problems associated with Sen's concerns regarding individuals or groups who have an inability to manage to desire adequately (Sen 1992) without then imposing paternalistic solutions. Many of the practicalities of handling communitarian claims remain to be resolved. At least, however, if there can be agreement that this paradigm is worthy of further development, then research at the empirical level can proceed. Most fundamentally this involves establishing how to set communitarian claims for health care for different groups in society.

CONCLUSION

There are a number of problems in both welfarism's and extra welfarism's treatment of equity in health care. As indicated in this chapter, many of these appear to be able to be overcome by adopting a communitarian approach to assessing claims.

Putting adequate flesh on the conceptual bones of this new approach remains to be done. It also remains to be seen whether it *can* be done. Particularly important here is the issue of eliciting community preferences and in turn communitarian preferences. These are matters which are particularly challenging for economists who have assumed to date that the only preferences that are relevant are individuals' preferences. It also requires a step back from the reductionism and quantification of economics.

ACKNOWLEDGEMENTS

We are grateful to the editors, Cam Donaldson, John Henderson and Kostas Mavromaras for comments on an earlier draft. GM is also grateful to the Health Department of Western Australia for financial support for his chair.

REFERENCES

Abelson J and Lomas J (1996) In search of informed input: a systematic approach to involving the public in community decision making. *Health Care Management Forum*, **9**(4), 48–52.

Arrow KJ (1963) Uncertainty and the welfare economics of medical care. *American Economic Review*, **53**, 941–973.

Aveneri S and de Shalit A (1992) Introduction. In S Aveneri and A de Shalit (Eds), *Communitarianism and Individualism*. Oxford University Press, Oxford.

Buchanan A and Mathieu D (1986) Philosophy and justice. In R Cohen (Ed.), *Justice: Views from the Social Sciences*. Plenum Press, New York.

Culyer AJ (1990) *Demand side socialism and health care*. Keynote Paper, the Second World Congress on Health Economics, University of Zurich, Zurich.

Donaldson C and Gerard K (1993) *Economics of Health Care Financing, The Visible Hand*. Macmillan, Basingstoke.

Garland MJ (2001) The Oregon Health Plan ten years later: ethical questions and political answers. In E Loewy and R Loewy (Eds), *Changing Health Care Systems from Ethical, Economic, and Cross Cultural Perspectives*. Kluwer Academic/Plenum Publishers, New York.

Houston S (2001) *Aboriginal Cultural Security*. Health Department of Western Australia, Perth.

Hunter DJ (1997) *Desperately Seeking Solutions: Rationing Health Care*. Longman, London.

Jan S, Mooney G, Ryan M, Bruggemann K and Alexander K (2000) The use of conjoint analysis to elicit community preferences in public health research: a case study of hospital services in South Australia. *Australian and New Zealand Journal of Public Health*, **24**(1), 64–70.

Klein R (1998) Puzzling out priorities. *British Medical Journal*, **317**, 959.

Leneghan J (1999) Involving the public in rationing decisions. The experience of citizens' juries. *Health Policy*, **49**, 45–61.

Margolis H (1982) *Selfishness, Altruism and Rationality*. Cambridge University Press, Cambridge.

McIntyre D and Gilson L (2000) Redressing dis-advantage: promoting vertical equity in South Africa. *Health Care Analysis*, **8**(3), 235–258.

Medical Council (2000) *Economics and Medicine: Bridging the Abyss*. Health Department of Western Australia, Perth.

Medical Council (2001) *What's Fair in Health Care*. Health Department of Western Australia, Perth.

Mooney G (1987) What does equity in health mean? *World Health Statistics Quarterly*, **40**(4), 296–303.

Mooney G (1994) *Key Issues in Health Economics*. Wheatsheaf, Hemel Hempstead.

Mooney G (1996) And now for vertical equity: some concerns arising from Aboriginal health in Australia. *Health Economics*, **5**(2), 99–104.

Mooney G (1998) 'Communitarian claims' as an ethical basis for allocating health care resources. *Social Science and Medicine*, **47**(9), 1171–1180.

Mooney G (2001) Communitarianism and health economics. In JB Davis (Ed.), *The Social Economics of Health Care*. Routledge, London.

Mooney G and Wiseman V (2000) A constitution for health services. *Journal of Health Services Research and Policy*, **4**(4), 195–196.

Mooney G, Jan S, Ryan M, Bruggemann K and Alexander K (1999) *What the community prefers, what it values, what health care it wants. A survey of South Australians*, SPHERe Report, SPHERe, Department of Public Health and Community Medicine, University of Sydney, Sydney.

Mueller DC (1989) *Public Choice*. Cambridge University Press, Cambridge.

Schokkaert E (1992) The economics of distributive justice. In KR Scherer (Ed.), *Justice: Interdisciplinary Perspectives*. Cambridge University Press, Cambridge.

Scottish Executive Health Department (1998) *Towards a Healthier Scotland*. SEHD, Edinburgh.

Scottish Executive Health Department (1999) *Fair Shares for All* (Arbuthnott Report). SEHD, Edinburgh.

Sen A (1977) Rational fools: a critique of the behavioural foundations of economic theory. *Philosophy and Public Affairs*, **6**, 317–344.

Sen A (1985) *Commodities and Capabilities*. North-Holland, Amsterdam.

Sen A (1992) *Inequality Reexamined*. Clarendon Press, Oxford.

Sen A (1993) Capability and wellbeing. In M Nussbaum and A Sen (Eds), *The Quality of Life*. Clarendon Press, Oxford.

Smith A (1759) *The Theory of Moral Sentiments*. Clarendon Press, Oxford.

Swedish Parliamentary Priorities Commission (1995) *Priorities and Health Care*. SOU, Stockholm.

Taylor C (1989) *Sources of the Self: the Making of the Modern Identity*. Cambridge University Press, Cambridge.

Vanberg VJ (1994) *Rules and Choice in Economics*. Routledge, London.

Wagstaff A and van Doorslaer E (1992) Equity in the finance of health care: some international comparisons. *Journal of Health Economics*, **11**, 361–387.

Williams A (1997) Intergenerational equity: an exploration of the 'fair innings' argument. *Health Economics*, **6**, 117–132.

Wiseman V (1999) Culture, self-rated health and resource allocation decision-making. *Health Care Analysis*, **7**(3), 207–223.

Wiseman V and Jan S (2000) Resource allocation within Australian Aboriginal communities: a program for implementing vertical equity. *Health Care Analysis*, **8**(3), 217–233.

objective function is health. Third, they do not allow for off creating. Fourth, operationalising across cases in different contexts... the notion of equity (it is) implicitly adopted... [text illegible]... position (in) that it is a principle of equity, that the preferences of the observer... as reflected in these weights can, however, also be used to assess... across groups. [text largely illegible]... respect the preferences of observers (it) represents... [text illegible]... they have some local variations within a framework of... health. See for example (Anand & Hanson 1997). It allows us to...that there is one particular set of a single system of values in applying equity weights.

[paragraph largely illegible]

A NEW PARADIGM

[text largely illegible] ... health ... equity ... (i) ... (ii) ... in deciding how the resources for equity in health care are to be allocated.[1] This new economics paradigm for equity in health care must be able to ... (i) ... value at the level of resource an equity goal that ... (ii) ... weights to be attached to ... individual benefits; (iii) ... based on the community view of their counterpreferential choices at the collective level (and) ... preferential at the community level; (iv) the principle that population groups treated inequitably should form the basis for how their inequities are then addressed; and (v) the idea that

---

[1] There is of course no reason why this approach need be restricted to health care. It could be used for most social goods, be handled in this way. It is likely however that for most goods the market will remain the method of choice for such allocations except where there is clear market failure as in the case of health care (personal communication, Mooney 2002).

12

Economics of Health and Health Improvement

ANNE LUDBROOK

Health Economics Research Unit, University of Aberdeen

DAVID COHEN

School of Care Sciences, University of Glamorgan

INTRODUCTION

The focus of most of the preceding chapters has been on the economics of health *care*, i.e. on the contribution that the formal health care sector makes to the production of health. It is evident, however, that health can be produced in many other ways. Indeed, the great health achievements of the 18th and 19th centuries were the result of public health measures such as improved sanitation, which had nothing to do with medical care. In the 21st century, incremental health gain through non-health care measures may again exceed the additional benefit achieved in the formal health care sector, particularly with respect to the persistent inequalities in health. For example, a recent review identified 34 evidence-based measures to reduce morbidity and mortality from heart disease and stroke, only eight of which involved use of the health care sector (Cochrane & Campbell Collaboration 2000).

The focus of this chapter is on the broader economics of health. In particular, it addresses some of the key questions that are posed for economic analysis when considering the impact of lifestyle and life circumstances on improving health. The importance of this area for health policy has grown over the past 25 years, largely due to recognition of the possibility that such interventions will have greater productivity at the margin than further investments in health care. It is also partly due to the recurrent interest in health inequalities and the role that lifestyle and life circumstances have in shaping these.

Advances in Health Economics. Edited by Anthony Scott, Alan Maynard and Robert Elliott.
© 2003 John Wiley & Sons, Ltd

The past 25 years have also seen a metamorphosis in health promotion. In its earlier years, the focus was on health education with reliance on the assumed links between increased knowledge, altered attitudes and changed behaviour which would reduce risk and ultimately lead to health gains. More recently, the focus has shifted away from its purely educational aspects, latterly with an emphasis on 'health development' which encompasses all aspects of health-affecting life circumstances.

Government attitudes to health have similarly changed during this period. Prevention and Health (Department of Health and Social Security 1977) was the first major policy statement in this area and its focus was on individual lifestyle factors. The 1979 Conservative government, with its ideology of personal responsibility and a reduced role for the state, further emphasized the role of lifestyle. Thus when the 1980 Black Report called for socio-economic solutions to the problems of inequalities in health between social classes (Townsend & Davidson 1990), the government's response was largely to ignore it.

Since then, the need to recognize the role of public policy and healthy surroundings in health improvement has crept back onto the agenda and was eventually incorporated into government strategy. Policy documents such as the Health of the Nation (Department of Health 1992) recognized that successive governments had been obsessed with health care *activity* rather than with health. The shift of focus from activity to *achievement* (in terms of health gain) recognized the limited role of the health care sector in producing health and brought a wide range of players from outside the formal health care sector into the health policy frame.

Since the election of a Labour government in 1997 this momentum towards a broader view of health and its determinants has continued. *Our Healthier Nation* (Department of Health 1999) adopted an even more holistic approach to health, acknowledging the effect of life circumstances on health and including an explicit commitment to tackling inequalities in health through inter-sectoral collaborative policies.

The next section of this chapter considers the scope of the area in general terms, highlighting the limited economic effort outside of health care. The third section reviews some of the more conventional economic approaches to studying the market for health-affecting goods. The importance of viewing the market for health-affecting goods within a more fundamental market for the commodity 'health' is considered, including conceptual models based on household production approaches to health creation and health-affecting factors that are outside of any individual's control. The fourth section reviews some of the more conventional economic evaluations of lifestyle interventions and the recent attempts to get economic evaluation built into the Health Impact Assessments of government policies. The chapter ends with a section on future challenges and an agenda for future research.

THE ECONOMICS OF HEALTH

Economics is a discipline whose well-developed tools can be, and have been, applied to a wide range of topics. Exactly what 'topic' health economics addresses, or more precisely how narrowly the topic should be defined, is still a contentious issue. At one extreme, Kielhorn and Graf von der Shulenburg (2000) have stated that '(h)ealth economics is a discipline that analyses the economic aspects of *the healthcare industry*, using methods and theories from economics . . . ' (p. 79, emphasis added). At the other extreme, Culyer (1981) has defined health economics as the application of the discipline and tools of economics to the subject matter of health. Several leading health economists have attempted to conceptualize the area diagrammatically. Williams (1987) produced a schematic structure of health economics under eight headings (Figure 12.1) and this has been widely used to encapsulate health economics.

Only two of these categories are specifically about health and these encompass the literature on health determinants and the measurement and valuation of health. However, there seems to be no intrinsic reason why health should not feature within the remaining categories, other than that they reflect the preoccupations of the time.

Health economics has from its outset been predominantly concerned with health care economics and the literature on health has been modest by comparison. A bibliography of 'health economics' publications in the English language up to 1974 yields just 21 references that fall outwith the area of health care (Culyer *et al.* 1977). More recently, Maynard and Kanavos (2000) reviewed publications in the two main health economics journals (*Health Economics* and the *Journal of Health Economics*) up to 1999 and found less than 20% of articles to be in the two categories relating primarily to health (Table 12.1).

Evans and Stoddart (1990) identified the gap between the developing research on the wider determinants of health and the focus of health policy primarily on issues related to the provision of health care. They argued that this was, at least in part, due to an absence of appropriate models to conceptualize the problems and they set out a comprehensive framework of the determinants of health (see Figure 12.2). Health care is shown to be one of many determinants that include social and physical environment, genetic endowment and individual behaviour. While health care is arguably a suitable, if narrow, topic for the application of economic methods and theories, it is evident from the Evans and Stoddart schema that it is by no means the sole producer of its principal output. *Health* economics ought therefore to address the complete range of determinants that produce (or reduce) that output.

A further point raised by Evans (1984) and by Evans and Stoddart (1990) is the need for a clear definition of the 'health' part of health economics, arguing that if health is synonymous with well-being or utility, then health economics

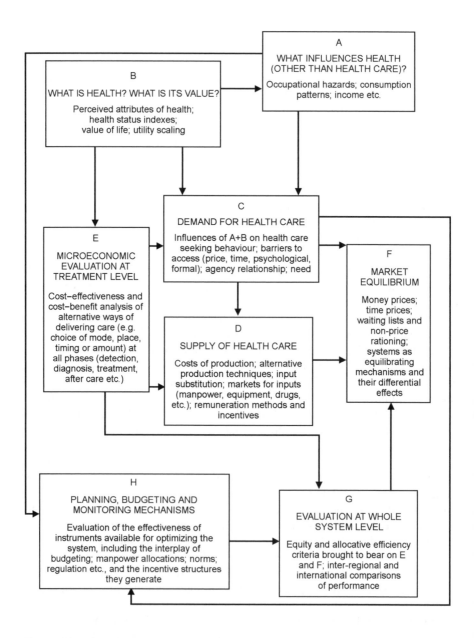

Figure 12.1 Health economics: structure of the area
Source: Maynard and Kanavos (2000), reproduced with permission of John Wiley & Sons, Limited, based on Williams (1987), reproduced with permission of Palgrave Macmillan

Table 12.1 Percentage of each article category with *Health Economics* and the *Journal of Health Economics* (1982–1999)

Article category	Total number of articles	Articles as % total
A. What influences health – other than health care?	84	11.4
B. What is health? What is its value?	57	7.8
C. Demand for health care	96	13.0
D. Supply of health care	152	20.7
E. Microeconomic evaluation at treatment level	108	14.7
F. Market equilibrium	57	7.8
G. Evaluation at whole system level	76	10.3
H. Planning, budgeting and monitoring mechanisms	90	12.3
Overview	16	2.2
TOTAL	736	100.0

Source: Maynard and Kanavos (2000).

becomes the economics of everything. There is a clear sense in which health is *not* synonymous with well-being. Trade-offs between health and other goods, services or activities can be observed on a daily basis. However, relatively little attention has been paid to the relationship between health (however perceived) and utility, and the resulting implications for individual behaviour. This is a key issue if health is to be the focus of interest.

There is a large and growing literature on the measurement and valuation of health, dominated by functional definitions and negative, disease-based models appropriate to decision-making within the health care sector (for a review see Dolan 2000). Some utility-based approaches are adopted, but broader measures of outcomes may be required to include other dimensions of health. In addition, many of the actions taken, both by individuals to improve their own health and by the state through a range of policies that affect the health of the population, also yield benefits over and above those directly from health improvements. The value of these actions must be based on the full range of benefits accrued. Difficulties in assessing the trade-offs (assuming they exist) between the utility from health and the utility from all other sources mean that it may not be possible to avoid 'the economics of everything' in this context. This is one of the important challenges to developing economic analysis.

MARKETS AND HEALTH

It has been argued that economists' focus on health care can at least in part be explained by the fact that health has no value in exchange; it is not traded and a market for health does not exist (McGuire *et al.* 1988). However, realism has

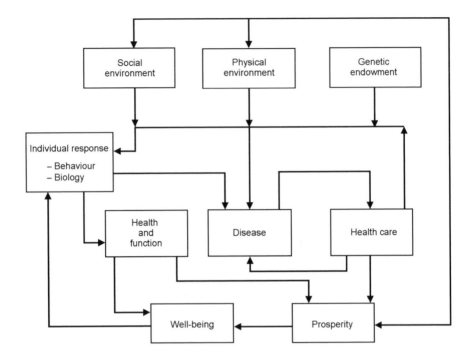

Figure 12.2 Determinants of health
Source: Reprinted from Evans and Stoddart 1990, with permission from Elsevier Science

never been a barrier to the economic paradigm and the absence of a market does not entirely explain the failure to analyse behaviour more often 'as if' a market did exist. Trade-offs involving risk were the basis of some of the early literature on value of life (e.g. Jones-Lee 1982; Mooney 1977), providing at least some basis for a value in exchange. Observed labour market behaviour provides a basis for valuing certain health states (see for example French & Dunlap 1998; Dobbs 1999; Sandy *et al.* 2001). Methods can be further developed to value attributes that are indirectly traded. (See for example Chapter 1 on contingent valuation methods and Chapter 2 on discrete choice experiments.)

THE MARKET FOR HEALTH-AFFECTING GOODS AND SERVICES

The behaviour of consumers and producers in the market for health can be approached in two basic ways. The first uses standard economic market theories applied to goods known to have an effect on health and for which markets exist. (The second approach, based on household production functions and demand for health, is considered in the next subsection). Interestingly, most of the work by health economists in this area has focused on goods that are detrimental to health such as tobacco, alcohol and illicit drugs. The research on smoking, alcohol and illicit drugs has recently been reviewed (Chaloupka & Warner 2000; Cook & Moore 2000; SBU 2001).

The literature on health-affecting goods includes policy-relevant analysis, such as the price elasticity of demand for cigarettes (e.g. Fujii 1980) and alcohol (e.g. Walsh 1982) and the consequences of price changes in terms of both consumption and revenue (e.g. Hu *et al.* 1995). Individual consumption behaviour has also been modelled, with attempts to account for features of health-affecting goods (mainly addiction) which make consumer behaviour different from 'normal' market goods (Becker & Murphy 1988; Jones 1999; Suranovic *et al.* 1999).

Little of this research has addressed the underlying demand for health that may influence individual behaviour. In particular, studies of individual commodities fail to take account of the consequences of changes in demand for other health-affecting commodities. Studies that have considered this issue have found both substitution effects and complementarity between such goods. For example, Dee (1999) found that higher cigarette taxes reduced both teenage smoking and the prevalence of teenage drinking and Farrelly *et al.* (2001) found similar effects for marijuana use. However, increasing the minimum age for legal drinking slightly reduced the prevalence of alcohol consumption and slightly increased the prevalence of marijuana consumption (DiNardo & Lemieux 2001). This suggests that there are different attributes relating to the consumption of different health-affecting goods.

DEMAND FOR THE FUNDAMENTAL COMMODITY 'HEALTH'

While all of the above relate to the market for health-affecting goods and services, none focus on the real commodity of interest – health. However, concentrating on the attributes of health and health-affecting goods may be a useful avenue to pursue. The origins of this approach lie with Becker (1964) who first proposed the concept of households being producers as well as consumers. Grossman (1972) applied this approach to health with a model in which individuals or households were both producers of health and consumers of health care. The Grossman model has been influential in conceptualizing the demand for health but it involves a number of assumptions about the relationship between utility and health.

Grossman argued that an individual's stock of health can yield two distinct types of utility; that from consumption (consuming yields more utility when healthy than when ill) and that from production (more health means more healthy time which means greater income and hence more consumption). This implies a contingency relationship in which health may be different from other arguments in the utility function.

The Grossman model makes no reference to other stocks (e.g. wealth or education), implying that the utility from greater health is independent of the individual's levels of these other stocks. Muurinen (1982) developed a Grossman-type model which included other stocks, and in which the rate at which individuals draw on their stock of health through consumption of hazardous goods depends on the relative size of the health stock compared with the others. In other words the utility from a change in health is not independent of other characteristics of the individual and individuals can trade health utility against other sources of utility.

The Grossman model also assumed that the utility from any increase in health stock is independent of its source. Ippolito (1981) showed that the demand for goods which increase risk is not independent of the *nature* of the hazard; in her case whether the hazard is constant (fixed probability of death per unit consumed) or cumulative. The importance of the nature of the hazard is also evident in the literature on risk (e.g. Mole 1976) that consistently shows that individuals will 'accept' higher risks that are under their own control (e.g. my decision to go hang gliding) than when imposed (e.g. environmental hazards). In these cases the utility from a change in health will not be independent of how it was brought about, suggesting that health improvements that arise from individual behaviour change may have a different role in the utility function from health improvements from external events such as improved housing or cleaner air. The degree of success in changing individual behaviour also appears to vary with the type of change being promoted (e.g. smoking compared with alcohol or dietary change). This suggests that more consideration needs to be given to the attributes of health that may vary in different settings, rather than treating it as a single entity.

While Grossman's landmark contribution has been influential in shaping the literature in this area, its focus was on the derived demand for health care. Grossman and Rand (1974) explored the relationship between prevention and cure in an extension to the demand for health model, and although explicitly recognizing that the consumption of goods other than health care affects the stock of health, they ruled out all types of joint production for the purposes of the model.

Subsequent literature has produced a number of developments and improvements, including further empirical estimates (Grossman 2000), but health care has tended to remain central to the analysis. As such, the 'market' analysis is only partial. Some factors that influence the efficiency of the household production function, such as education and income, have been included but this particular approach cannot encompass all the health-affecting activities in which individuals engage (Muurinen 1982). What remains less explored is the extent to which the demand for *other* health-affecting goods, particularly those whose consumption *reduces* the risk of illness or injury, can be explained by demand for health models.

CONCEPTUAL MODELS OF HEALTH-AFFECTING BEHAVIOUR

Health-affecting behaviour can be considered in terms of the demand for health-affecting (both positive and negative) goods. A major difficulty of conceptualizing health-affecting behaviour within a demand for health framework is that health-affecting goods run along a continuum from those demanded solely for their effects on health (vitamin supplements) to those which may have only incidental effects on health and may be demanded for reasons unrelated to health (exercise).

Cohen and Mooney (1984) developed a taxonomy of health-affecting goods and services which led to a conceptual model of preventive behaviour (Cohen 1984) based on the demand for prevention goods and hazard goods. The essence of the 'utility model of preventive behaviour' was that much of the demand for prevention goods, defined as goods whose consumption reduces the risk of future ill-health, could be perceived as being derived from the demand for health. On the other hand, the demand for hazard goods, defined as goods whose consumption increases the risk of future ill-health, would have to be viewed differently. On the assumption that better health is preferred to worse health, hazard goods will only be demanded if they yield positive utility from other attributes of the good.

Both prevention goods and hazard goods were thus seen as potentially yielding utility from two sources: the use value of the good (utility-in-use) and the knowledge that consuming the good alters risk (utility-in-anticipation). In the case of prevention goods, utility-in-use could be negative, as would be the case in all health care, or positive. For hazard goods, utility-in-use would have to be positive. Utility-in-anticipation would be positive for prevention goods from the knowledge that risk is reduced and negative for hazard goods from the knowledge that risk is increased. The demand for any prevention or hazard good is thus dependent on the relationship between the sum of the two types of utility and its price. Examination of the factors which influence utility-in-anticipation, which *inter alia* include the individual's own time preference rate and degree of risk aversion, leads to policy implications which suggest a move away from traditional health education as a means of altering preventive behaviour.

Other expected utility models have been developed in the context of insurance. Ehrlich and Becker (1972) proposed that, in response to uncertainty, self-protection and self-insurance activities were alternatives to market-based insurance offering monetary compensation. Self-protection is consistent with primary prevention and self-insurance with secondary prevention. Interactions between preventive and curative services have also been explored (Nordquist & Wu 1976; Phelps 1978; Kenkel 1994).

PRODUCING HEALTH – WIDER DETERMINANTS OF HEALTH

While health can be regarded as a fundamental commodity produced by consumers it is clear that any individual's level of health stock and its rate of depreciation are affected by numerous factors outside of the individual's control (see Figure 12.2). The health determinants model can be seen as the basis for considering the production of health from a societal perspective. While some factors may have to be taken as given (e.g. health endowment at birth, genetic disposition) others can be influenced by government policies which are not solely aimed at health issues but which may nevertheless have major impacts on health. The extent to which such health effects are yielded only 'incidentally' will vary greatly between these non-health care policies.

At one extreme are the broad policies to manage the macro-economy. Although these are clearly pursued for reasons that are not health-related they may nonetheless have significant health impacts. For example, some research findings suggest a relationship between unemployment and health (Brenner 1973, Moser et al. 1984), although other research has cast some doubts on whether the evidence supports this (Gravelle & Simpson 1981; McAvinchey 1982; Wagstaff, 1985). If true, then any government measure aimed at reducing unemployment can at the same time be regarded as health policy. Other policies may be explicitly addressing issues related to the wider determinants of health but little is known about their effects on health. For example, there are consistent findings of a strong association between inequalities in health and inequalities in income (van Doorslaer et al. 1997; Benzeval & Judge 2001), with some studies addressing the issue of causality (Ettner 1996). However, specific research on the impact of poverty reduction measures is lacking. Evidence reviewed for the Acheson Report identified only one trial relating to income support, and the health outcome employed – effect on low birth-weight – was relatively short-term (Kehrer & Wolin 1979; Department of Health 1998).

Other, more specific government measures may have an even stronger but still incidental effect on health. For example, while housing policy is primarily concerned with improving living conditions *per se*, such improvement can also have significant impacts on health; for example where damp conditions lead to respiratory diseases or hazards in the home have high risks of accidents. Again, whilst there is an established link between poor housing and poor health, there is only limited evidence of the impact of specific interventions (Thomson et al. 2002). Other policies such as environmental protection may have a more explicit health-producing aim, while others such as occupational health and safety will be specifically aimed at health.

Overall, evidence of the potential health improvement to be derived from tackling the wider determinants of health remains only potential. The marginal productivity of these measures as compared to the marginal productivity of health care is largely unknown (Cochrane & Campbell Collaboration 2000). Some evaluations of specific interventions have been undertaken and these are reviewed briefly in the next section, but these reveal rather patchy progress in measuring the productivity of policy measures.

ECONOMIC EVALUATION OF HEALTH-AFFECTING INTERVENTIONS

Standard economic evaluation methods have been applied in the health-affecting area to a broad range of lifestyle interventions either directly (e.g. Godfrey 1994) or as risk factors for specific diseases (e.g. Baxter *et al.* 1997). It is beyond the scope of the present chapter to provide a comprehensive review and indeed the number of economic appraisals in this area is becoming so large that an overall review is becoming increasingly difficult.

It should be noted, though, that economic evaluations of health-affecting behaviour have been biased towards evaluations which come close to a treatment model, particularly in the case of smoking cessation (e.g. Nielsen & Fiore 2000). With respect to treating alcohol and drug abuse, a recent review identified only 24 economic evaluations (of 1200 studies which included discussion of costs) and judged half of these to be of low scientific quality (SBU 2001). There are fewer studies in other lifestyle areas such as dietary interventions (Pritchard *et al.* 1999) or exercise (Sevick *et al.* 2000). The relative lack of *economic* evaluations in some areas may be related to the lack of good quality evaluations on which to base such analysis.

Economic evaluations of broader health promotion programmes are less common. Mass media advertising campaigns for quitting or prevention of smoking have been evaluated (Ratcliffe *et al.* 1997). Health education approaches or health promotion interventions have been used to reduce cardiovascular risk factors, either on their own (Salkeld *et al.* 1997) or in association with risk factors for other diseases (Fries & McShane 1998).

Some of the economic studies on specific policies, such as tobacco and alcohol taxation, have been referred to earlier. An additional area of anti-smoking legislation that has been assessed is the impact of advertising bans or controls. Few economic studies have been carried out relating to other aspects of government legislation and these tend to be evaluations of enforcement issues such as drink-driving.

In recent years there has also been a growing recognition of the need to evaluate the health effects of non-health policies. Guidance on how government departments and other public sector agencies should appraise health impacts of broader public policy was first set out in 1995. Further guidance on Health Impact Assessment (HIA) has since been published (Cabinet Office 1999) which recommends rigorous economic appraisal and is largely consistent with Treasury guidance on appraisal and evaluation (the 'Green Book'), as well as guidance published by different government departments. Guidance on how to perform such rigorous economic appraisals is now widely available.

However, outwith government departments the main practitioners of HIA have largely eschewed this approach. In particular, the emphasis placed on considering the objectives that are being addressed, and the *alternative* policy options that are available to achieve them, has been largely ignored. Widely followed guidelines for HIA have been developed that concentrate on the health impacts of single projects, and how these might be ameliorated (if negative) or enhanced (if positive) (Scott-Samuel et al. 1998). Partly because of the rejection of the overtly quantitative approach of economic appraisal and evaluation, many HIA studies fail to consider the evidence of effectiveness and cost-effectiveness.

Similar to the way in which economic evaluations of lifestyle issues have focused on behaviours which increase risk, HIA has also focused on policy factors which have a detrimental effect on health. Less is known about the comparative effectiveness of policies that improve health and/or reduce inequalities in health. Such evidence is undoubtedly difficult to assemble and liable to be incomplete. A recent compilation of the evidence from systematic reviews of research relevant to the 'wider public health' agenda reveals the extent of the gaps in current knowledge (Cochrane & Campbell Collaboration 2000). In respect of interventions to reduce health inequalities, the Acheson Report (Department of Health 1998) and the work of its associated evaluation group (Macintyre et al. 2001) have highlighted the paucity of the evidence base.

There are also issues in evaluation which arise from the nature of some of the programmes being evaluated. A recent consultation document (Department of Health 2001) identifies both eradication of child poverty and improving educational opportunities as part of a wide-ranging strategy for improving the health of children in low-income families. These provide examples of the type of policy initiative that pose particular challenges in carrying out evaluation to provide robust evidence of cost-effectiveness for policy-making.

These interventions have potential macroeconomic implications, whereas economic evaluation is essentially a microeconomic tool. Some of the impacts will be very long term and the nature of the interventions is such that direct comparisons between interventions and the *status quo* are not feasible. This is not to say that evaluation cannot or should not be carried out, but rather that the standard methods of economic evaluation need to be adapted and developed. This will be necessary in order to measure and compare the impact of such policies with interventions that have more direct effects and shorter time scales. The problems of conducting economic evaluation in the broader health field are shared with other social welfare programmes (Sefton et al. 2002).

FUTURE CHALLENGES AND AN AGENDA FOR RESEARCH

The focus of health economics has been predominantly on health care and there is considerable scope for a shift of research effort towards health, particularly in the light of increasing policy interest in the wider determinants of health. More research on health implies more research addressing some of the conceptual challenges of such a shift in paradigm, as well as more evaluation research on the cost-effectiveness of health improvement interventions.

The main conceptual themes that emerge relate to the definition, measurement and valuation of health, the relationship between health and other sources of utility and the demand for and production of health. In all these areas, it seems important to accept that health may not be a single entity and that consideration of attributes of health may provide more promising opportunities for research. One of the potential uses of discrete choice experiments may be to establish willingness to pay values for programmes (Ryan 1999) or to provide trade-off values for different attributes. In the context of evaluations, these methods may avoid the need to explore definitions of health and utility in any depth. However, such explorations could forward an understanding of individual behaviour and motivation in respect of demand for health and health-affecting goods, where the contribution of economics to date has been minimal.

In empirical work, there has been a bias towards exploiting existing data; hence the emphasis on issues such as tobacco and alcohol, where market data are available. In posing broader questions, researchers will have to consider other sources of secondary data as well as the possibility of generating primary data from questionnaires and choice experiments. Economic evaluation studies have clearly been circumscribed by the availability of effectiveness evidence but, again, it is possible that evidence does not need to be limited to experimental interventions but other sources of longitudinal or cross-sectional data can be exploited. The use of routinely collected data sets is increasingly being seen as a way of reducing current reliance on randomized controlled trials (Raftery et al. 2002).

Recently, Edwards (2001) reviewed four 'visions of the future of health economics' by established leaders in the field: Williams (1993), Phelps (1995), Maynard and Kanavos (2000) and Fuchs (2000). She concluded that all four visions, and their associated research agendas, are almost exclusively focused on health care rather than health (with Fuchs to a lesser extent).

Edwards (2001) presents an alternative paradigm which builds on Williams' schematic presentation of the main element in health economics (Williams 1987). In particular Williams' two core elements 'demand for health care' and 'supply of health care' are replaced with 'health of society' and 'health of the individual' to emphasize that health rather than health care ought to be seen as the relevant social want. She also adds an element 'macroeconomic evaluation of public policy and health' to allow cross-sectoral programme budgeting and marginal analysis of prevention to be considered within the paradigm. If health economics is to include everything relevant to the supply and demand for health, then Edwards' view possibly represents a more appropriate framework.

This approach raises some interesting challenges for the direction of future research. For example, within the conventional health care paradigm, advances in the area of measuring and valuing health states (a single element of the Williams schema) has mainly been driven by the need for an outcome measure to assess the cost-effectiveness of different health care interventions. Thus the debate about quality adjusted life years (QALYs) has to address the issue of whose values ought to be used. The Edwards' paradigm on the other hand, with its separation of 'health of society' from 'health of the citizen', provides an opportunity for a focus on individuals' decisions about health-enhancing and health-harming behaviour which is based solely on individuals' valuations. Similarly, the addition of the element 'macroeconomic evaluation of public policy and health' emphasizes the importance of non-health policies on the health of individuals and society.

The future research agenda should encompass theoretical developments in understanding the 'market' for health, particularly the demand for health and the way in which health enters the individual's utility function, as well as research in policy appraisal and economic evaluation. Discrete choice experiment methods offer opportunities to explore the trade-offs between health and other attributes of health-affecting goods and may provide insights into the value attached to health. Better methods of evaluation need to be developed and applied. These should include exploring the use of secondary data sets to assess the impact of policies on health and not simply to establish statistical associations between health and life circumstances. In particular, longitudinal data sets could be used in the framework of before and after studies. More generally, however, a change in focus towards *health* economics rather than *health care* economics is required.

ACKNOWLEDGEMENTS

The authors are grateful to Janelle Seymour and Steve Birch for helpful comments on an earlier draft and to all the participants at the HERU workshop. Core funding to HERU from the Chief Scientist Office, Scottish

Executive Health Department is gratefully acknowledged. All opinions expressed are the responsibility of the authors.

REFERENCES

Baxter T, Milner P, Wilson K, Leaf M, Nicholl J, Freeman J and Cooper N (1997) A cost effective, community based heart health promotion project in England: prospective comparative study. *British Medical Journal*, **315**, 582–585.

Becker G (1964) *Human Capital*. Columbia University Press, New York.

Becker GS and Murphy KM (1988) A theory of rational addiction. *Journal of Political Economy*, **96**(4), 675–700.

Benzeval M and Judge K (2001) Income and health: the time dimension. *Social Science and Medicine*, **52**, 1371–1390.

Brenner MH (1973) Fetal, infant, and maternal mortality during periods of economic instability. *International Journal of Health Services*, **3**, 145–159.

Cabinet Office (1999) *Modernising Government Cm4310*. The Stationery Office, London.

Chaloupka FJ and Warner KE (2000) The economics of smoking. In AJ Culyer and JP Newhouse (Eds), *Handbook of Health Economics Volume 1B*. Elsevier, Amsterdam.

Cochrane and Campbell Collaboration (2000) *Evidence from systematic reviews of research relevant to implementing the wider public health agenda*. NHS Centre for Reviews and Dissemination, http://www.york.ac.uk/inst/crd/wph.htm.

Cohen D (1984) Utility model of preventive behaviour. *Journal of Epidemiology and Community Health*, **36**, 61–65.

Cohen D and Mooney G (1984) Prevention goods and hazard goods: a taxonomy. *Scottish Journal of Political Economy*, **31**(1), 92–99.

Cook PJ and Moore MJ (2000) Alcohol. In AJ Culyer and JP Newhouse (Eds), *Handbook of Health Economics Volume 1B*. Elsevier, Amsterdam.

Culyer AJ (1981) Health, economics and health economics. In J van der Gaag and M Perlman (Eds), *Health, Economics and Health Economics*. North-Holland, Amsterdam.

Culyer AJ, Wiseman J and Walker A (1977) *An Annotated Bibliography of Health Economics*. Martin Robertson, London.

Dee TS (1999) The complementarity of teen smoking and drinking. *Journal of Health Economics*, **18**(6), 769–793.

Department of Health and Social Security (1977) *Prevention and Health*. HMSO, London.

Department of Health (1992) *The Health of the Nation. A Strategy for England*. HMSO, London.

Department of Health (1998) *Independent Inquiry into Inequalities in Health Report* (The Acheson Report).

Department of Health (1999) *Saving Lives: Our Healthier Nation Cm 4386*. The Stationery Office, London.

Department of Health (2001) *Tackling Health Inequalities. Consultation on a plan for delivery*. Department of Health, London.

DiNardo J and Lemieux T (2001) Alcohol, marijuana, and American youth: the unintended consequences of government regulation. *Journal of Health Economics*, **20**(6), 991–1010.

Dobbs IM (1999) Compensating wage differentials and the value of life. *Economics Letters*, **63**, 103–109.

Dolan P (2000) The measurement of health related quality of life for use in resource allocation decision in health care. In AJ Culyer and JP Newhouse (Eds), *Handbook of Health Economics Volume 1B*. Elsevier, Amsterdam.

Edwards RT (2001) Paradigms and research programmes: is it time to move from health care economics to health economics? *Health Economics*, **10**(7), 635–650.

Ehrlich I and Becker G (1972) Market insurance, self-insurance and self-protection. *Journal of Political Economy*, **80**, 623–649.

Ettner SL (1996) New evidence on the relationship between income and health. *Journal of Health Economics*, **15**(1), 67–85.

Evans RG (1984) *Strained Mercy. The Economics of Canadian Health Care*. Butterworths, Toronto.

Evans RG and Stoddart GL (1990) Producing health, consuming health care. *Social Science and Medicine*, **31**(12), 1347–1363.

Farrelly MC, Bray JW, Zarkin GA and Wendling BW (2001) The joint demand for cigarettes and marijuana: evidence from the National Household Surveys on Drug Abuse. *Journal of Health Economics*, **20**(1), 51–68.

French MT and Dunlap LJ (1998) Compensating wage differentials for job stress. *Applied Economics*, **30**, 1067–1075.

Fries JF and McShane D (1998) Reducing need and demand for medical services in high-risk persons: a health education approach. *Western Journal of Medicine*, **169**(4), 201–207.

Fuchs VR (2000) The future of health economics. *Journal of Health Economics*, **19**(2), 141–157.

Fujii ET (1980) The demand for cigarettes: further empirical evidence and its implications for public policy. *Applied Economics*, **12**, 479–489.

Godfrey C (1994) Assessing the cost-effectiveness of alcohol services. *Journal of Mental Health*, **2**, 3–21.

Gravelle HSE and Simpson P (1981) Mortality and unemployment: a critique of Brenner's time series analysis. *Lancet*, **ii**, 275–279.

Grossman M (1972) On the concept of health capital and the demand for health. *Journal of Political Economy*, **80**, 223–255.

Grossman M (2000) The human capital model. In AJ Culyer and JP Newhouse (Eds), *Handbook of Health Economics Volume 1B*. Elsevier, Amsterdam.

Grossman M and Rand E (1974) Consumer incentives for health services in chronic illness. In SJ Mushkin (Ed.), *Consumer Incentives for Health Care*. Millbank Memorial Fund, New York.

Hu T-W, Ren Q-F, Keeler TE and Bartlett J (1995) The demand for cigarettes in California and behavioural risk factors. *Health Economics*, **4**(1), 7–14.

Ippolito PM (1981) Information and the life cycle consumption of hazardous goods. *Economic Inquiry*, **19**, 529–558.

Jones AM (1999) Adjustment costs, withdrawal effects, and cigarette addiction. *Journal of Health Economics*, **18**(1), 125–137.

Jones-Lee MW (Ed.) (1982) *The Value of Life and Safety*. North-Holland, Amsterdam.

Kehrer B and Wolin V (1979) Impact of income maintenance on low birthweight; evidence from the Gary experiment. *Journal of Human Resources*, **14**, 434–462.

Kenkel DS (1994) The demand for preventive medical care. *Applied Economics*, **26**, 313–325.

Kielhorn A and Graf von der Shulenburg JM (2000) *The Health Economics Handbook*. Adis International, Chester.

Macintyre S, Chalmers I, Horton R and Smith R (2001) Using evidence to inform health policy: case study. *British Medical Journal*, **322**, 222–225.

Maynard A and Kanavos P (2000) Health economics: and evolving paradigm. *Health Economics*, **9**, 183–190.

McAvinchey ID (1982) *Unemployment and mortality: some aspects of the Scottish case, 1950–1978*. Health Economics Research Unit Discussion Paper No. 10/82, University of Aberdeen, Aberdeen.

McGuire A, Henderson J and Mooney G (1988) *The Economics of Health Care. An Introductory Text*. Routledge and Kegan Paul, London.

Mole RH (1976) Accepting risks for other people. *Proceedings of the Royal Society of Medicine*, **69**, 107–113.

Mooney GH (1977) *The Valuation of Human Life*. Macmillan, London.

Moser KA, Fox AJ and Jones DR (1984) Unemployment and mortality in the OPCS longitudinal study. *Lancet*, **ii**, 324–329.

Muurinen JM (1982) Demand for health: a generalised Grossman model. *Journal of Health Economics*, **1**, 5–28.

Nielsen K and Fiore MC (2000) Cost–benefit analysis of sustained-release buprorion, nicotine patch, or both for smoking cessation. *Preventive Medicine*, **30**, 209–216.

Nordquist G and Wu SY (1976) The joint demand for health insurance and preventive medicine. In R Rosett (Ed.), *The Role of Health Insurance in the Health Services Sector*. National Bureau of Economic Research, New York.

Phelps CE (1978) Illness, prevention and medical insurance. *Journal of Human Resources*, **13**, 183–207.

Phelps CE (1995) Perspectives in health economics. *Health Economics*, **4**(5), 335–353.

Pritchard DA, Hyndman J and Taba F (1999) Nutritional counselling in general practice: a cost-effectiveness analysis. *Journal of Epidemiology and Community Health*, **53**, 311–316.

Raftery J, Roderick P and Stevens A (2002) *Potential use of routine databases in health technology assessment*. NHS R&D HTA Programme Report, in press.

Ratcliffe J, Cairns J and Platt S (1997) Cost effectiveness of a mass media-led anti-smoking campaign in Scotland. *Tobacco Control*, **6**(2), 104–110.

Ryan M (1999) Using conjoint analysis to take account of patient preferences and go beyond health outcomes: an application to in vitro fertilisation. *Social Science and Medicine*, **48**, 535–546.

Salkeld G, Phongsavan P, Oldenburg B, Johannesson M, Convery P, Graham-Clarke P, Walker S and Shaw J (1997) The cost-effectiveness of a cardiovascular risk reduction program in general practice. *Health Policy*, **41**, 105–119.

Sandy R, Elliott RF, Siebert WS and Wei X (2001) Measurement error and the effects of unions on the compensating differentials for fatal workplace risks. *Journal of Risk and Uncertainty*, **23**(1), 33–56.

SBU (Swedish Council on Technology Assessment in Health Care) (2001) *Treatment of alcohol and drug abuse – an evidence-based review*. Stockholm.

Scott-Samuel A, Birley M and Arden K (1998) *The Merseyside Guidelines for Health Impact Assessment*. Merseyside Health Impact Assessment Steering Group, Liverpool. www.liv.ac.uk/~mhb/publicat/merseygui/ (accessed 20/12/00).

Sefton T, Byford S, McDaid D, Hills J and Knapp M (2002) *Making the most of it. Economic evaluation in the social welfare field*. Joseph Rowntree Foundation and York Publishing Services, York.

Sevick MA, Dunn AL, Morrow MS, Marcus BH, Chen GJ and Blair SN (2000) Cost-effectiveness of lifestyle and structured exercise interventions in sedentary adults: results of project ACTIVE. *American Journal of Preventive Medicine*, **19**(1), 1–8.

Suranovic SM, Goldfarb RS and Leonard TC (1999) An economic theory of cigarette addiction. *Journal of Health Economics*, **18**(1), 1–29.

Thomson H, Petticrew M and Morrison D (2002) *Housing Improvement and Health Gain: A summary and systematic review*. MRC Social and Public Health Sciences Unit Occasional Paper No. 5, University of Glasgow.

Townsend P and Davidson N (1990) The Black Report (edited version). In P Townsend, N Davidson and M Whitehead (Eds), *Inequalities in Health*. Penguin Books, London.

van Doorslaer E, Wagstaff A, Bleichrodt H, Calonge S, Gerdtham UG, Gerfin M, Geurts J, Gross L, Häkkinen U, Leu RE, O'Donnell O, Propper C, Puffer F, Rodriguez M, Sundberg G and Winkelhake O (1997) Income related inequalities in health: some international comparisons. *Journal of Health Economics*, **16**, 93–112.

Wagstaff A (1985) Time-series analysis of the relationship between unemployment and mortality: a survey of econometric critiques and replications of Brenner's studies. *Social Science and Medicine*, **21**, 985–996.

Walsh BM (1982) The demand for alcohol in the UK: a comment. *Journal of Industrial Economics*, **30**, 439–446.

Williams A (1987) Health economics: the cheerful face of the dismal science? In A Williams (Ed.), *Health and Economics*. Macmillan, Basingstoke, pp. 1–11.

Williams A (1993) Priorities and research strategy in health economics for the 1990s. *Health Economics*, **2**(4), 295–302.

Index

Note. Abbreviations used in the index are: DCEs = discrete choice experiments; GPs = general practitioners; WTP = willingness to pay.